Liz Earle
SKIN
SECRETS

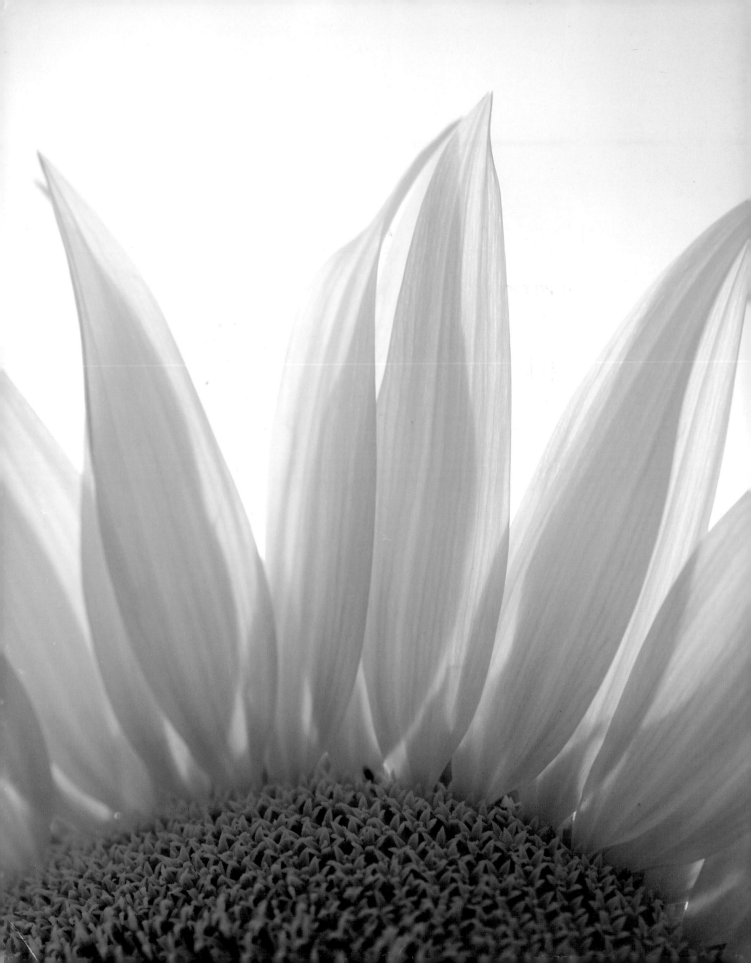

Liz Earle

SKIN SECRETS

Discover healthy, beautiful skin

Liz Earle

Special photography by Patrick Drummond and Kate Whitaker

Illustrations by Kathy Wyatt

Kyle Books

Contents

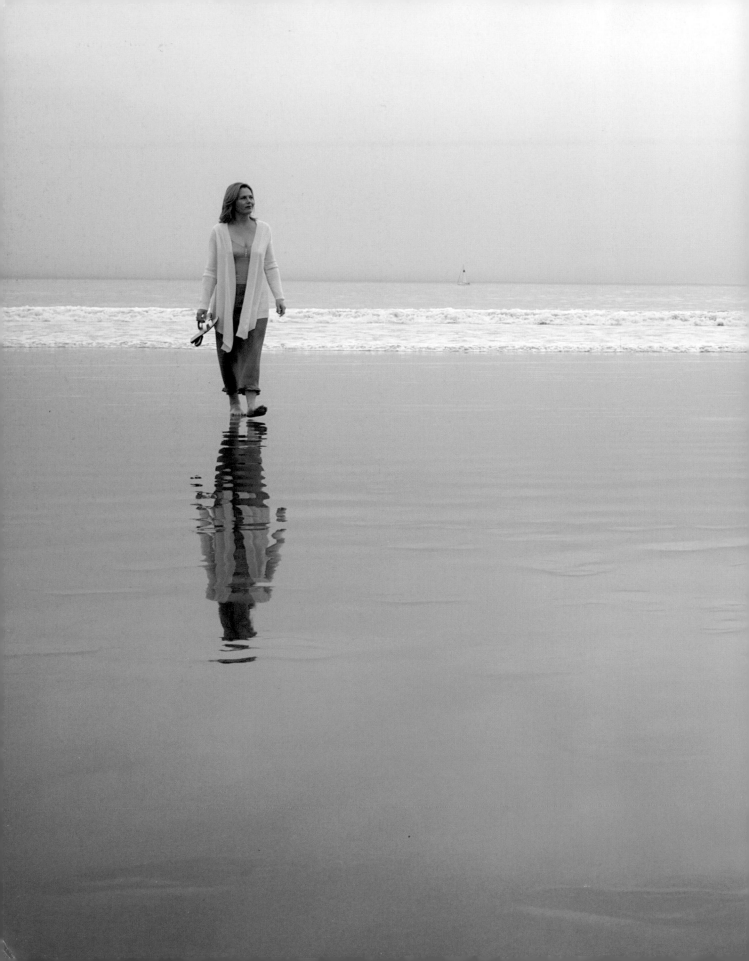

Stress

When we're happy, healthy and relaxed, our skin invariably is too. Research is now showing that psychological stress damages skin in a similar way to external stressors such as environmental pollutants. When we're anxious or under pressure, our two adrenal glands, which sit on top of each kidney, release the 'fight or flight' hormones – adrenaline and cortisol. In ancient times, when humans had to run away from mountain lions or warring tribes, this mechanism was vital to increase the sugar levels in your blood, so we had the energy to escape. Nowadays, we don't work off stress by running for miles and if too many stress hormones are chasing round the body because of worry, not enough sleep, too much work or emotional trauma, it can be destructive. When our blood sugar rises, insulin – the hormone that processes sugar – is produced; this, in turn, triggers inflammatory chemicals in the cells, which are linked to spots, acne and many other skin problems (more on page 118). It's also known that cortisol blocks the formation of collagen, the main protein which provides a network of support for your skin, making it toned and bouncy. High levels of cortisol also affect the immune cells in the epidermis, disrupting the skin barrier and weakening the skin's defences against UV light, other pollutants and infections. Additionally, psychological stress may cause a direct reaction on the facial skin by triggering the release of brain chemicals called neuropeptides into the nerve endings. One neuropeptide, known as Substance P, can provoke the production of more sebum and inflammatory chemicals called cytokines, both of which can lead to acne.

Sleep

My mother used to tell me that an hour's sleep before midnight is worth two after. (What that means, in fact, is that you shouldn't get overtired.) Beauty sleep is well named: it is an irreplaceable part of skincare. After a good night's rest, wrinkles and furrows are ironed out – but it's not clear whether this is due to switching off from waking pressures plus a temporary accumulation of fluid (which plumps out wrinkles but can also make eyes and tissue puffy) or to a speeding up of skin cell production at night, which some research suggests. Interestingly, it may not be sleep itself that produces the result, but a state the British Association of Dermatologists calls 'relaxed wakefulness', which suggests that meditation, prayer or any peaceful activity will benefit our skin, too.

Night is certainly an ideal time for the skin to absorb moisture and nutrients. The temperature of the body is higher too, increasing blood flow to the skin – hence the rosy glow when we awake. The sleep hormone melatonin itself acts as an indirect antioxidant, by increasing the activity of the main antioxidant enzymes and other chemicals that protect cells against free-radical damage. Conversely, lack of sleep leaves skin looking tired and washed out and triggers dark circles underneath your eyes. Sleep deprivation weakens the immune system, which may trigger disorders such as eczema. A bad night's sleep also increases the production of the stress hormone cortisol, which can last all day, leading to the effects of stress.

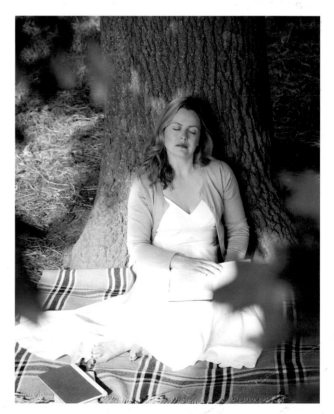

How our skin works

Our skin is far more than just an outer cosmetic wrapping – it's a highly sophisticated mechanism and the largest organ of the body.

The skin is not simply a waterproof mac for the body: it is an organ with a nervous system which monitors outside assaults such as cold, heat and environmental toxins, and internal assaults such as stress or illness. The skin 'talks' to the brain. It's said that the skin is the body's 'brain on the outside'.

Skin is similar to an eggshell. The outside protects us from the elements, repels bugs, parasites and other invaders, and protects our internal organs against injury and the sun. Crucially, it also keeps water inside. Our bodies are over 70 per cent fluid, so if we weren't safely encased in our skins we would dry out and deflate like frogs or jellyfish when they leave a watery environment. Skin is such a smart mechanism, however, that it lets us perspire to keep our internal body temperature at a safe level. That, incidentally, is why scientists believe we lost most of our body hair: hairless skin allows sweat to evaporate quickly so it cools the body more efficiently. (The thatch on our heads is there to protect our brains from the sun.) But our skin does far more: it's our interface with the world. Think about it: you touch a baby's skin and register the softness through your own. When you're embarrassed, your skin flushes. It warns us of pain, heat and cold and, of course, betrays our age, both in its degree of elasticity and thickness. Skin is unique, remarkable and, to me, completely fascinating.

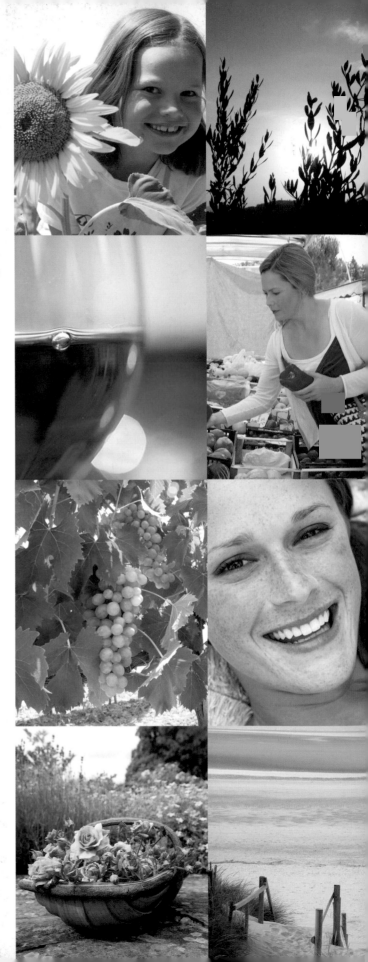

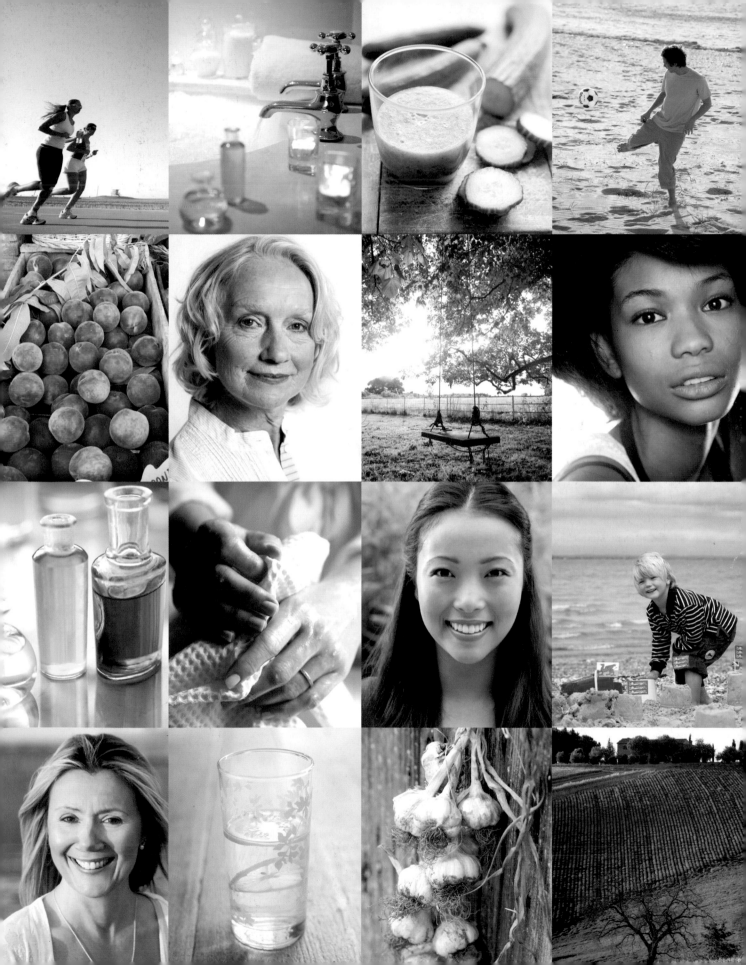

The structure of skin

Imagine a slightly flat cream cake slice with three main layers sandwiched together and lots of thinner ones within them. Our skin is a bit like that. The main layers are the epidermis – the top part we see and touch, then the dermis, and underneath that the subcutaneous fatty layer.

Epidermis:

The top layer or epidermis (derma means 'skin' in Greek – hence a dermatologist is a skin specialist – and epi means 'over') is a light-reflecting, translucent (like frosted glass) covering for the body. It's amazingly thin for something so tough – about 1mm (1000 micrometres) over most of the body, but at its thinnest on areas such as eyelids it is only about 0.05mm (50 micrometres), and at its thickest on the soles of our feet or palms of our hands it is 1.5mm (1500 micrometres). It contains no blood vessels and is nourished from capillaries in the top layer of the dermis below.

All day, every day, skin cells (keratinocytes) are being born, developing and dying in the five levels of the epidermis. The cells begin life at the basal layer of the epidermis, then move up through the five levels, changing shape and developing all the time. By the time they reach the surface, or horny layer, the cells have died, flattened and are being sloughed off – a process called exfoliation or desquamation – and more 'daughter' cells are on their way up. The whole process takes 26–42 days, according to American dermatologist Leslie Baumann. Over our adult life, the process gradually slows and dead cells linger on the surface, which is why we notice duller, less radiant skin in older people.

The structure of the epidermis

Bottom of the epidermis:

1. Stratum basale or basal layer: The skin cell factory, where millions of new, column-shaped cells are produced 24/7 from stem cells. As soon as they are formed, they're pushed up through the other skin layers by the constant production of new cells beneath them. Melanocytes, or pigmentation cells, start here too. The amount of melanin you produce controls skin colour, how much we tan, hair colour, and also helps protect your skin against sunlight. The skin's immune cells (Langerhans cells) originate here, to act as one of our first defences against invading bugs. Nerve endings reach up from the basal layer to the surface layer, where they respond to touch, heat, cold and pain.

2. Stratum spinosum or spinous layer: The cells, now irregular in shape and multi-sided, start to produce keratin, the main protein which makes up skin, nails and hair. Lipids (fats) appear, also making their way up to the surface to form the skin barrier.

3. Stratum granulosum: The busy shop floor of the skin factory, where keratin and lipids, including moisture-retaining ceramides, are developing further.

4. Stratum lucidum: Often referred to as part of the next layer the stratum corneum, this layer exists only on your palms and soles. The cells flatten and clump together to produce an extra layer of protection where they encounter most friction.

5. Stratum corneum or horny layer: the top surface layer – like the icing on the cream cake slice. The cells here, called corneocytes, are now 25 to 30 layers of dead, flattened discs, tightly packed and cemented with lipids (fats) and proteins as a brick wall-like barrier. Its thickness varies enormously, from 0.01mm (10 micrometres) in fragile areas such as the eyelid (making them very sensitive to harsh detergents such as soap or SLS) to 0.1mm (100 micrometres) on the soles of the feet.

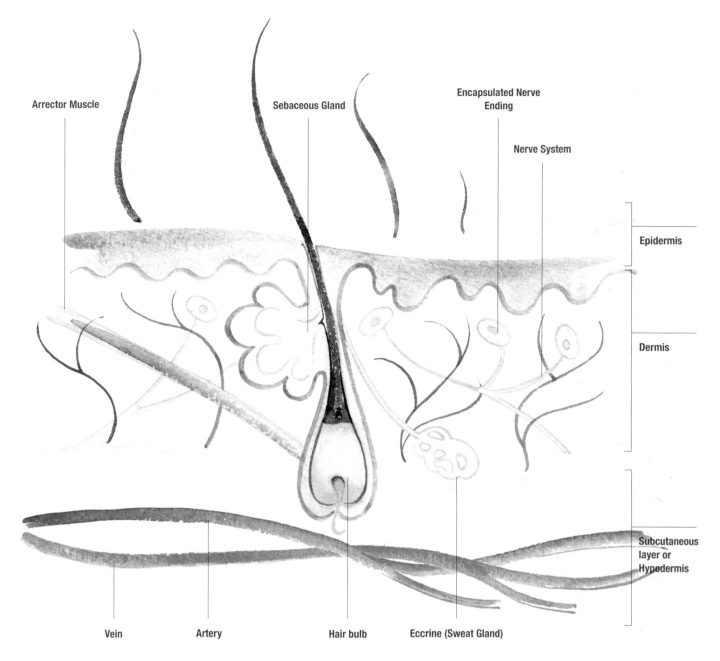

Arrector Muscle

Sebaceous Gland

Encapsulated Nerve Ending

Nerve System

Epidermis

Dermis

Subcutaneous layer or Hypodermis

Vein   **Artery**   **Hair bulb**   **Eccrine (Sweat Gland)**

Although the corneocytes are technically dead by this stage, they contain many chemicals that enable this dynamic barrier to respond to, and protect us from, the environment and prevent the loss of water. One important group of chemicals are called Natural Moisturising Factor (NMF). NMF acts like a magnet for water, attracting it into the corneocytes so they swell up, preventing the formation of cracks in between them. This is why healthy skin is so smooth and shiny. In dry skin, however, there are reduced levels of NMF within the corneocytes and small cracks can develop – that's the reason dry skin feels rough and loses

its healthy lustre. Good moisturisers contain constituents such as plant oils, glycerin and hyaluronic acid that mimic the deficient NMF and so help rehydrate the corneocytes, restoring the smooth, healthy skin surface.

If the stratum corneum barrier is damaged, it allows 'trans-epidermal water loss' (TEWL). Bad burns, for instance, cause massive water loss – but this loss also increases with dermatitis, eczema, psoriasis, etc. High TEWL is linked to raised permeability, making it easier for external irritants to enter the epidermis, resulting in increased sensitivity and dry skin. Moisturisers work mainly by reducing TEWL.

pH and the acid mantle of the skin

The term pH stands for 'potential of hydrogen' which measures the hydrogen concentration of any substance: we also know it as the 'acid/alkaline balance'. It is graded from 0 to 14, with 0 being the most acid, 14 the most alkaline, and 7 being the neutral, or mid-point. The stomach has a pH of around 1, because you need stomach acid to break down food. The protective layer on the skin surface known as the 'acid mantle' (a mix of sebum and sweat) has a mildly acidic pH, which helps to kill bacteria and fungi: it's thought to function optimally at the skin's 'normal' pH of 5.5. Many skin products are labelled 'pH balanced', meaning they have been formulated to have a pH close to 5.5. Soapy water has an alkaline pH of around 9.5 and, if you overwash the face with strongly alkaline soaps or cleansers, the acid mantle becomes more alkaline and the skin is more prone to infection and damage.

Dermis:

This middle layer is connected to the epidermis by the 'basement membrane', a soft, pliable but strong layer of tissue. The dermis is thicker than the epidermis, again varying over different parts of the body from about 0.3mm on your eyelids up to 3mm or more on your back. The thickness doubles between the ages of three and seven, and again at puberty.

The dermis is made up mostly of bundles of collagen – one of the strongest natural proteins, which gives skin elasticity and bounce – held together with fibres of another protein, elastin. It's the breakdown of collagen and elastin, owing to sunlight and other external problems, as well as internal factors – notably, stress – plus the natural changes of ageing, that cause skin to lose its tone and start to sag. All around the collagen and elastin is hyaluronic acid, a sticky, slippery substance (because it attracts and holds water), which is essential for skin moisture.

As you can see in the drawing on the previous page, this layer has lots of sweat glands and follicles, nerves and also blood vessels, which supply oxygen to the epidermis and take away waste products.

Sweat glands

Sweat is vital for regulating body temperature and keeping the skin moist. As you perspire, the moisture on your body evaporates and cools the skin, regulating the temperature of the whole body. These glands are also activated when you're nervous or frightened – as in the sweaty-palm response. You have between 2–4 million sweat glands, capable of producing up to a litre of sweat an hour, even more when in a hot climate.

There are two types of sweat gland, eccrine and apocrine, both of which begin life in the dermis. The eccrine glands, which are responsible for most output and are found all over the body, are long, hollow tubes with a coil at the bottom where the mixture of water and salts which makes up sweat is produced. It then flows up the tube to the opening (pore) on the skin's surface.

Apocrine glands are similar, but they're attached to hair follicles, mainly under the armpits and in the genital area. Although they produce much less sweat, it's more concentrated and contains proteins and fats which are responsible for your individual smell. Apocrine sweat glands can be turned on or off by the autonomic nervous system, but this operates as a whole so when one gland is activated, all glands spring into action. The eccrine glands are more precisely controlled and different parts of the body work independently, which is why your palms can sweat when you're extremely nervous while your face remains dry.

Follicles

Tube-like structures called follicles – some containing a hair, some empty – originate in the bottom of the dermis, extending up to the skin surface, where you see them as pores.

Branching off the follicles are grape-like clusters of sebaceous (oil) glands, which produce the oily substance known as sebum. Sebum makes its way into the follicle and then up to the skin surface, where it mixes with sweat to become what's known as the 'acid mantle' (see above).

Each hair follicle has small muscle fibres called arrector

pili attached to it, which contract when you're cold or frightened causing the follicle to protrude slightly above the surface. This is technically called piloerection – more commonly known as 'goose bumps'. Stem cells located around the arrector pili are mainly responsible for our hair growth and the average growth rate for a healthy head of hair is around 0.4mm (400 micrometres) a day.

Subcutaneous layer or hypodermis:

At the bottom of the imaginary cream cake slice is a cushion of fat, called the subcutaneous layer, which is filled with adipose (fat-filled) cells, blood vessels and nerves. This varies in thickness: on your bottom, for instance, it's several millimetres thick, but entirely absent on eyelids, and thinner on the neck. This layer helps plump up the skin, keep you warm, protect your bones and acts as a useful energy reserve tank in times of famine. It's also involved in synthesising vitamin D from the sun, which is vital for healthy bones and teeth, boosting the immune system and reducing inflammation in the body.

Normally, the skin is quite loosely attached to muscle and bone with connective tissue, but if the fatty layer over-expands (because you put on weight, for example), then the fibres in the connective tissue are pulled tight, resulting in the mattress-like dimpling of our favourite skin villain, cellulite.

The dermis is made up mostly of bundles of collagen – one of the strongest natural proteins, which gives skin elasticity and bounce

How to find your skin type

The 'T' zone runs across the forehead, down the nose to the chin, forming the letter T

Before you decide how to treat your skin, it's essential to know its strengths and weaknesses, then choose products and treatments accordingly.

As you've seen, your skin is very much influenced by many external (and internal) factors. If you've been blessed with an unblemished complexion, live a stress-free life and possess peerless genes, then your skin is probably perfect and needs little more than a wash with a cloth. For the rest of us mortals, using plant-based skincare makes visible improvements. Fortunately, almost all of us can balance, normalise and improve our skin with appropriate plant-based skincare and some simple lifestyle shifts. I've even witnessed those with naturally good skin being truly amazed at how much *better* their skin looks and feels with judicious care. Formulations such as sunscreens, moisturisers, eye creams and serums also help to delay the ageing process and keep skin younger looking than if they are not used. When choosing what to use on your skin though, it's important to know your skin type. When Kim Buckland and I set up Liz Earle Beauty Co. in 1995, we focused on two simple skincare regimes: one for dry skins – like mine – and the other for normal and combination skins, such as Kim's. We later expanded this to include oily skins, for our daughters, and very dry/mature skins, for our mothers (and now ourselves…). Thousands of loyal customers worldwide tell us that this approach works – and so I'm confident it will work for you too.

NB: there is a different set of skin types for categorising your 'burn risk' – how vulnerable you are to sunlight – which I explain on page 109.

Oily skin

Has large pores and shiny skin, especially on the T-zone (forehead, nose and chin); skin tends to be thicker, with rough, irregular texture and colouring; is prone to blackheads and spots; is very common in teenagers and young adults, rare after the age of 35.

Normal and combination skin

Normal skin has medium-size pores; looks clear, with even colour; feels soft and bouncy to the touch; isn't tight or greasy; doesn't feel uncomfortable or irritated; isn't essentially prone to blackheads or spots.

Combination skin: The only difference between this and normal skin is that combination skin, which the majority of women are thought to have, has an oilier T-zone and may be prone to breakouts there; cheeks tend to be normal, possibly a little on the dry side, especially in winter.

Dry skin

Has fine pores; feels flaky or rough, sometimes with red patches; feels tight and sometimes irritated after washing, especially if you have used soaps or been in a dry atmosphere for some time; fine lines develop early around the eye area.

Very dry/mature skin

Has fine pores; feels tight; has visible wrinkles and broken capillaries; skin is slacker on the cheeks and jawline; may have a leathery texture on very thin areas.

Sensitive skin

Has fine pores; tends to be thin and is prone to broken capillaries; flushes easily; is inclined to rashes and irritation; can extend to any skin type, including oily, but mostly affects people who are prone to allergic conditions, in particular, eczema, asthma and hay fever.

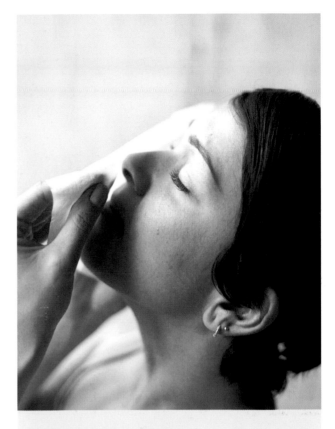

Testing skin type

Most people know what skin type they are, but if you can't decide, either talk to a skincare consultant at your favourite store, or try this simple test:

❋ Remove any make-up, rinse your face with water, pat it dry with a clean towel and leave for 1 hour.

❋ Place a single layer of white tissue (peel apart a tissue and it will give you two or three thin layers) over your face and press it over the surface, pushing it into the corners and crevices.

❋ Leave it for a few minutes, then lift off and inspect the result.

❋ **Oily skin:** the tissue will stick to sebum, pick up oily spots and become translucent.

❋ **Normal/combination skin:** it will stick only to your T-zone.

❋ **Dry/very dry skin:** the paper won't stick to any area of your face as you have very little sebum.

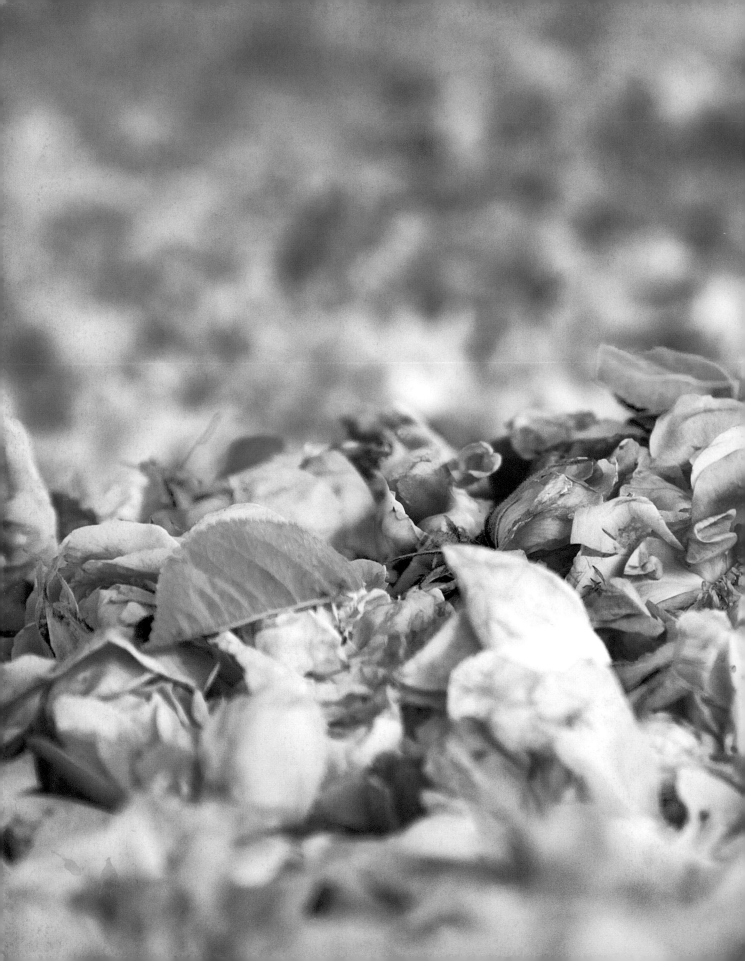

Chapter Two

PLANTS THAT LOVE YOUR SKIN

Botanical ingredients have kept skin beautiful
and healthy for thousands of years. I am a big
fan of their plumping, soothing and smoothing
qualities. Here are some of my favourites.

Plant oils

Pure natural plant oils are used in skincare
for their therapeutic effects and because
they're so easily absorbed into the upper
layers, where they get to work beautifying
our skin.

Argan oil

(*Argania spinosa*)

One of my 'secret' ingredients for helping to restore a youthful glow is Moroccan argan oil, so precious the locals call it 'liquid gold'.

Around the coastal town of Essaouira in Morocco, the one place in the world where the argan trees grow, you might see a goat or three balanced precariously on the branches. The goats love the nuts, which look like a cross between a walnut and an almond, as much as the Berber women who gather them.

When I first visited this sub-Saharan desert region to research argan oil for its skin-repairing properties, I was struck by just how smooth the Berber women's skins were, despite the fierce climate in which they live. They extract the oil from the nuts by hand and lavish it onto their skin, hair, nails – and even their babies. I bought two bottles

from the local women's cooperative in this Muslim community: one went to our labs to be analysed and the other made its way to my fridge. It's delicious used as the Moroccans do, drizzled over salads and couscous.

The oil proved to be remarkably high in antioxidant vitamin E (alpha tocopherol), which protects and repairs skin cells, and also phytosterols (plant fats). The combination of these phytosterols is unique to the argan tree and includes relatively rare types. More research (I practically moved into the British Library) revealed clinical studies with claims that argan speeded wound-healing, skin cell stimulation and regeneration: these were particularly linked to two compounds – alpha-spinasterol and delta-7 stigmasterol.

French scientists have also demonstrated the oil's ability to boost moisture within the skin, as well as stimulating oxygenation between the cells. It also helps neutralise free radicals, the molecules that break down the structure of skin cells, causing the signs of premature ageing and, potentially, skin cancer.

The coastal town of Essaouira in Morocco is the one place in the world where argan trees grow

Borage

(*Borago officinalis*)

Borage seed oil is a rich source of two essential fatty acids called linoleic acid (LA) and gamma-linolenic acid (GLA) and it's particularly good for people with dry, flaky complexions. My own love affair with plant oils began more than 20 years ago when I took a supplement of borage seed oil (sometimes called 'starflower' oil), which helped to clear my own eczema.

Extensive research has confirmed that a daily dose of GLA (in the form of borage seed oil or evening primrose seed oil) quietens inflamed skin – and I still take it today if my skin shows signs of a flare-up. In addition, applying borage seed oil topically starts to moisturise skin immediately and visibly.

Herbalists have long used borage for sore or inflamed skin, including eczema and other chronic skin conditions. Studies show that skin creams containing borage seed oil significantly decrease skin roughness and water loss through the skin. I regard it as a key 'naturally active' ingredient and use it liberally throughout many of the Liz Earle nourishing skin creams for face and body.

Borage is an easy plant to grow. Its pretty, star-shaped flowers, which range from bright blue to purple as the blooms go over, contrast with the soldier-straight stems covered with stiff, white, prickly hairs. The amount of GLA extracted from the seeds varies according to where the borage is grown. In the UK, for example, Yorkshire farms have a higher GLA yield than borage grown in Kent.

Herbalists have long used borage for sore or inflamed skin, including eczema and other chronic skin conditions

Passionflower extract has been documented for its calming, sedative action for more than 200 years

rows of small amber bottles, which are sold at roadside beauty kiosks to use as an emollient skin and hair oil.

The flowers are succeeded by large, purpley-orange fruit. These passion fruit are delicious to eat (cut them in half and scoop out the pulp with a teaspoon) and packed with seeds which yield the skin-cherishing, pale yellow oil. As well as vitamin E and trace minerals, it has an extraordinarily high content of linoleic acid, one of the essential fatty acids that is quickly absorbed by the skin and helps reduce water loss, thereby restoring elasticity.

There are some 400 types of passionflower, mostly originating from tropical America, with some species coming from Asia, Australia and the Polynesian islands. The passionflower was probably brought into Europe by Spanish explorers who had found it in South America in the mid to late sixteenth century, where it was widely used by the native Indians. Passionflower extract has been documented for its calming, sedative action for over 200 years (often in combination with valerian root and melissa – commonly known as lemon balm), and these days is recognised by regulatory bodies, including the European Scientific Cooperative on Phytotherapy.

Passionflower
(*Passiflora incarnata*)

This vine, which will climb up to 4–5m, is one of the most beautiful and colourful medicinal plants, with its stunning purple-tinged petals. The dense corona of filaments, or threads, around the central stamens seemed, to sixteenth-century Italians, to resemble a crown of thorns – which led to its common name 'fior della passione' or flower of the Passion (of Christ) and later to its botanical equivalent *passiflora*.

I discovered the oil in Kenya, where the lovely flowers grow like weeds; the pure passion fruit seed oil is found in

Avocado

(*Persea gratissima*)

Delicious to eat (and so good for you – and your skin), the creamy-textured, greeny-yellow flesh of avocados yields an unctuous oil that I love to use in skincare for its super-moisturising properties. As well as vitamin E (also traces of B vitamins and beta-carotene in unrefined versions), avocados contain omega-9 essential fatty acid, a little omega-6, plus chlorophyll, which may help regenerate skin cells. The rich oil, which is very easily absorbed, is also high in plant sterols, which may help to reduce age spots and to heal sun damage and scars. Avocado oil is especially useful for those with dry or mature skins. It works very well for most with sensitive skin, also eczema or psoriasis. I like to see it as an ingredient in soaps, massage oil and facial masks for its emollient properties. Avocado oil can be found in supermarkets and is a fabulous addition to salad dressing.

The wonderfully light texture
means it's easily absorbed into the
uppermost level of the skin

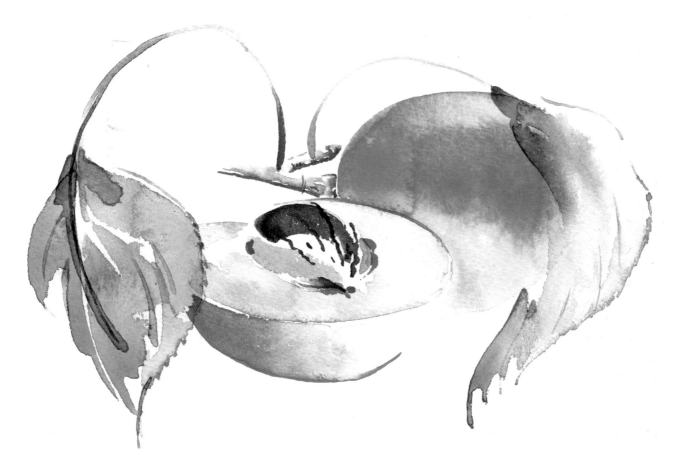

Apricot

(*Prunus armeniaca*)

Apricots, which come from the same *prunus* genus as peaches, plums and almonds, have been cultivated in their birthplace in the mountains of north China for four thousand years. Trade and military expeditions by plant-loving generals such as Alexander the Great brought them to the Middle East and onto Greece and Italy in about the first century BC, where they are now cultivated.

The kernels are crushed to yield between 40–50 per cent pure oil, which contains much the same array of fatty acids as sweet almond and peach kernel. The wonderfully light texture means it's easily absorbed into the uppermost level of the skin: dry, mature, sensitive and inflamed skins benefit most. Apricot oil also has very little odour, so it's an ideal base for facial and body massage oil blends. For a bath oil, add a drop or two of your favourite essential oil to one tablespoonful of apricot (or peach kernel) oil and mix with your fingertip before adding to a full tub.

Sweet almond

(*Prunus amygdalus dulcis*)

Sweet almonds are incredibly generous with their oil, giving nearly half their weight when the shelled nuts (in fact, the seed) are pressed. Almond oil, which contains essential fatty acids, vitamin E and traces of B vitamins, has long been used topically: John Gerard, the eminent sixteenth-century herbalist, wrote, 'The oil of almonds makes smooth the hands and face of delicate persons, and cleanseth the skin from all spots and pimples.' It's certainly accepted today that sweet almond oil is very mild and non-irritating, so is particularly suitable for sensitive and/or allergic skins and is often used by aromatherapists as a base for massage oil. Many natural health professionals recommend it for people with acne, too, because it is lightweight and non-comedogenic, so doesn't clog pores.

It's also a wonderful oil to use on your hair, for lustre and gloss. You can use it neat to strengthen nails (the Empress

Are nut oils allergenic?

Many ask whether nut oils can affect allergy sufferers. The eight major allergens include peanuts and tree nuts. Researchers at Southampton University carried out trials on 60 adults allergic to peanuts – which actually aren't nuts, but legumes (like peas). Each adult was fed refined and un-refined peanut oil. None of the 60 people tested had a reaction to the refined oil, which removes the proteins that can cause allergic reactions in sensitive people. Six people had a reaction to the unrefined oil. The researchers concluded that the sample of 60 people proves to a very high level of statistical probability that refined peanut oil is safe for peanut-allergic people. The same is believed to be true of real nut oils, such as almond. (We always use refined nut oils in Liz Earle formulations, for just this reason.) However, I always recommend patch testing new products of any kind – and particularly those that contain any traces of nut oil – on a small area of skin for 24 hours, before applying more widely.

Josephine lavished 'crème amande' on her hands), to soften the skin on your face and body and in the bath. It's an excellent carrier for essential oils: beauties in ancient Egypt blended a few drops of frankincense essential oil with almond oil as an 'anti-wrinkle' formula.

And, of course, almonds as food are a marvellous source of vegetable protein, providing significant amounts of the essential amino-acids that the body can't make, plus useful minerals (more on eating nuts on page 145).

Rosehip oil

(*Rosa rubiginosa*)

Rosehips remind me of my home in the southwest of England, as our farm hedgerows are dotted with these vibrant orangey-red fruits from late autumn onwards. This luxurious oil is pressed from the seeds and is one of my all-time favourites for its visibly regenerative properties. It's probably the most effective plant oil for skin repair and restoration, which makes it perfect for older skins.

Rosehip oil is rich in antioxidants – notably vitamin E – and essential fatty acids. It also contains vitamin A in the form of trans-retinoic acid, which helps remove the top dead layer of skin cells, exposing the fresher, brighter skin underneath by natural exfoliation.

Clinical studies have proven its ability to soften scars, reduce 'age' pigmentation spots and patches (which also tend to affect women in pregnancy), and improve the appearance of fine surface lines.

A trial of 141 patients with scarring and dried or very wrinkled skin used a high percentage (26 per cent) of rosehip oil added to a cream base. The 123 patients with scarring greatly benefited, as did the patients with leathery skin; the five patients with keloid (raised) scars also showed surface improvement. This effect is thought to be due to interesting compounds called phyto- (plant) sterols, which are fats, or lipids.

We blend it into the Liz Earle facial oil (Superskin Concentrate) for overnight nourishment, or you can use it neat on specific problem areas, such as scarring. The older the scar, the longer it will take to work but, applied daily, you should see a difference after about a month.

> This luxurious oil is one of my all-time favourites for its visibly regenerative properties

Essential oils

Romantically described as the 'life-force' of a plant, these highly fragrant liquids are known by chemists as volatile oils. Each carries a distinctive scent – the essence of the plant.

Neroli
(*Citrus aurantium amara*)

This deliciously fragrant oil, a personal favourite that I've used in many skincare formulations, is distilled from the blossom of the orange tree (*Citrus aurantium amara*), which grows mainly around the Mediterranean in Spain, Morocco, Italy and Tunisia. The orange tree is one of the most versatile sources of fragrant oils: orange oil is expressed from the peel; petitgrain is distilled from the twigs and leaves, and neroli – the most precious – from the tiny white blossoms. Touching the delicate petals damages the fragile oil glands, so the flowers are shaken from the trees and collected in huge sheets first thing in the morning, before the valuable oil starts to evaporate in the heat of the sun. The flowers are taken straight to the still and processed within hours. Neroli was named after a princess of Nerola in Italy, who liked to wear it as a perfume and made it fashionable as a scent. It combines fresh sharp citrus notes

Neroli was named after a princess of Nerola in Italy, who liked to wear it as a perfume

with sweet warm florals, an unusual odour profile which makes it one of the classic ingredients in eaux de colognes, such as the now cult 4711. Diluted into creams and massage oils, neroli is relatively well tolerated on the skin and has a toning, balancing effect. Aromatherapists often use the soothing aroma of neroli to help relieve fear, anxiety and shock.

Lavender (*Lavandula angustifolia*)

When French physician René-Maurice Gattefossé burnt his hand in a lab experiment, he thrust it into a vat of lavender oil. Amazed at how quickly his hand recovered, he was inspired to record the healing properties of many other essential oils, and coined the term 'aromatherapy'. His book, *The Practice of Aromatherapy,* is the standard work on the subject.

The sweet-scented, mauve-flowered bush has a long history as a medicinal herb. It grows wild around the Mediterranean – thriving in even the poorest soil: the name comes from the Latin 'lavare', meaning to wash, suggesting the Romans used it to fragrance the water they washed in. It was part of their herbal pharmacopoeia, grown wherever they set up camp (alongside rosemary, parsley, fennel and borage). Perhaps they used it, as herbalist John Parkinson suggested in 1640, for 'griefes and pains of the head and brain'. Modern science testifies to lavender's powers to help rest and relaxation (tuck a sprig into your pillow case) as well as to help alleviate headaches – massage a few drops into the temples.

The oil is also strongly antiseptic and I keep a small bottle in the kitchen to use neat on small burns and grazes, cuts and insect stings. I also like to sprinkle a few drops into a warm bath, and mix five drops in a 100ml spray bottle of pure water for a refreshing summer after-sun skin spritz.

Lavandula angustifolia is said to produce the best quality medicinal oil and the Liz Earle supplies are grown in the Sault region of France. Once it's been cut and distilled, we store it for up to 18 months to let the fragrance mature, much like a fine wine.

Mint
(*Mentha x piperita* and *Mentha spicata*)

Many species of mint have been used to produce essential oils but the two most in favour now are the sharply-fragrant peppermint (*Mentha x piperita*) and softer-scented spearmint (*Mentha spicata*), the type most used in cooking.

The main constituents in peppermint are menthol-type compounds, best known for their ability to create a cooling effect on the skin, while spearmint is rich in carvones, which produce a chilling effect almost like a local anaesthetic.

While we all know about using mint in cooking, toothpaste and chewing gum, we may be less familiar with its use in skincare. But that cool-as-a-mountain-stream freshness gives a zing to toners and any product designed to revive and stimulate the skin. It also helps brighten the complexion by encouraging a rosy glow. Preparations containing peppermint oil have been found to help relieve the scaly skin linked to conditions such as acne and also dermatitis, making it useful in shampoo.

In aromatherapy, it's used to ease muscular pains and headaches; in fact it makes an appearance in stick form as a non-drug panacea for tension headaches.

Tea tree oil is a fabulous first-aid remedy for insect bites, spots, boils and minor wounds

Tea tree
(*Melaleuca alternifolia*)

In 1770 the explorer Captain James Cook, who was travelling north along the coast of New South Wales, met native Australians (Aborigines) who prepared a spicy tea from this small tree or shrub – and so the name was born. The folk history of the leaves' healing properties goes back beyond records, but the oil was not commonly used until Australian chemist Dr Arthur Penfold published papers on its anti-microbial activity in the 1920s and 30s. This gave rise to the commercial tea tree oil industry. Demand waned after the Second World War, presumably with the development of effective antibiotics, but revived in the 1970s, with the re-emergence of interest in traditional and natural medicine.

Nearly 100 chemical compounds have been identified in tea tree oil; the most important appears to be an anti-bacterial called terpinen-4-ol, which makes up about 40 per cent of the oil. It's been shown to treat moderate acne as effectively as benzoyl peroxide, although more slowly, and anecdotal reports suggest it can help eradicate the tiny white bumps of the increasingly common, contagious virus *molluscum contagiosum* (often found in children), for which conventional medicine has no answers. It also has antifungal activity and is known to treat dandruff and seborrheic dermatitis effectively.

Tea tree oil is used for insect bites, spots, boils and minor wounds. It can also help ease ear infections and bee stings. Laboratory studies report that tea tree oil has shown activity against MRSA. A bottle of this multi-purpose oil is a must for any natural medicine chest. NB: it should never be taken by mouth and may sometimes cause contact dermatitis in sensitive people when applied topically.

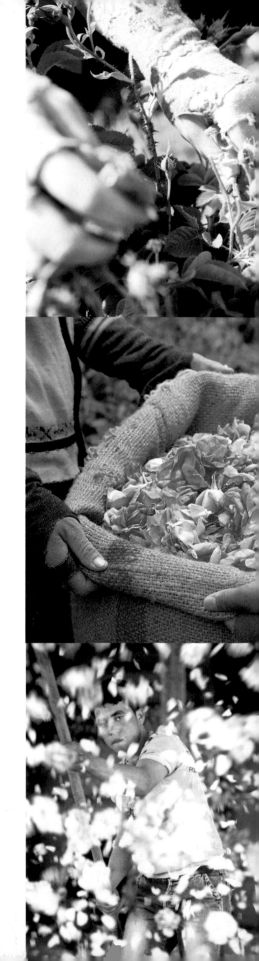

Rose

(*Rosa centifolia* and *Rosa damascena*)

This is one of my favourite essential oils for its divine scent and gentle skin-toning properties. Pure rose oil is one of the most precious essential oils, as it takes a full metric tonne of the fragile blooms to produce just 200ml. There are two main types of rose from which the volatile fragrance oils are extracted: firstly, *Rosa centifolia* (or more accurately, a hybrid of *Rosa centifolia* and *Rosa gallica*), which is also commonly known as cabbage rose, or *Rose de mai*; there is also *Rosa damascena*, or damask rose, the variety usually favoured by perfumiers (it's pictured here).

I've visited both the south of France and Turkey to take part in the rose harvest. Each morning the growers gather early, before the sun rises and starts to evaporate the valuable volatile oils. It's a family affair, as children join parents and grandparents to ensure each bloom is carefully hand-plucked and placed into hessian sacks (plastic would contaminate the petals). It's a magical time, with the scent of roses filling the air as literally millions of flowerheads are loaded onto tractors, spread out to dry on warehouse floors, then tipped into huge vats to begin distillation with water or steam to produce the oil. Solvent extraction – the alternative processing method – gives 'rose concrete', which is further processed with alcohol to produce 'rose absolute'. The quantity of oil is variable; an abundance of flowers won't necessarily yield the greatest oil content, whereas an apparent paucity of blooms may produce much more, as quantity depends on how enriched the petals are.

Rose is a complex oil, with over 300 chemical constituents, including the important perfumery constituents called citronellol, geraniol, nerol and phenylethyl alcohol, plus minor ones which impart subtly differing aromas. It has both skin-calming and mood-uplifting properties and is a very special addition to massage blends for face and body.

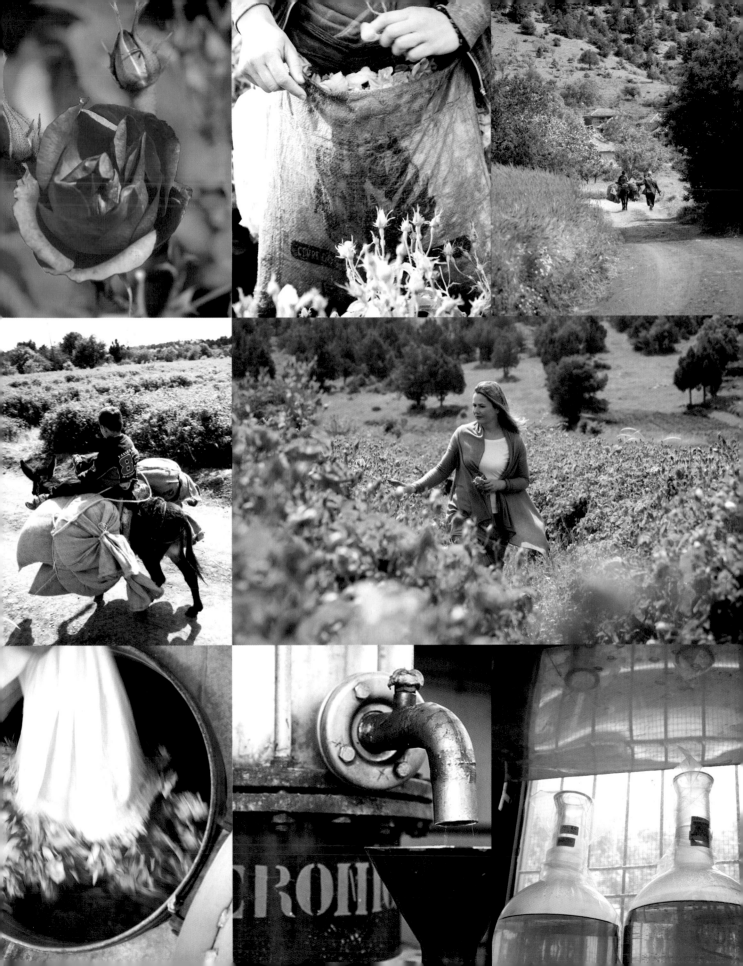

Wonder ingredients

Many plant extracts, juices, waxes and butters yield unique skin benefits only found in botany.

Aloe vera
(*Aloe barbadensis*)

This African native, which also grows obligingly in a pot on a windowsill, is one of the oldest known medicinal plants. Break open a leaf and the juicy, gel-like sap that seeps out has proved to be a dramatically effective healer of wounds and burns (including sunburn), speeding up the rate of healing and reducing the risk of infection. Aloe juice contains salicylic acid, both antibacterial and anti-inflammatory, which can help soothe inflamed skin conditions, such as dermatitis. Unlike its conventional rival, hydrocortisone, which treats inflammation but blocks wound healing – aloe actively helps skin to repair by stimulating cell production and increasing the collagen content of the damaged tissue. Aloe is also reported to increase elastin fibre which, with collagen, forms the matrix underpinning the skin and giving it tone.

This succulent plant with long, mottled, spiky leaves, which looks cactus-like but, in fact, belongs to the Asphodelaceae family, was depicted on Egyptian temple friezes as early as 4,000BC. Cleopatra is reputed to have used aloe as a beauty staple and it's been shown to reduce the formation of 'age' or 'liver' spots, due to substances called anthraquinones, which help block the production of melanin (the brown pigment).

Taken internally, the gel helps inflammatory bowel disease, while 'bitter aloes' (dried liquid from the leaves) stimulates digestion and, in higher doses, relives constipation.

Shea butter

(*Butyrospermum parkii*, *Vitellaria nilotica* or *V. paradoxa*)

This fabulously effective, totally natural moisturiser is indispensable for nourishing and soothing dry and inflamed skin; it's also used in haircare products. Shea butter (or shea nut butter) is a creamy-coloured, natural (and edible) fat extracted from nuts inside the crushed fruit of the shea tree. It's a similar skincare ingredient to cocoa butter, another pod 'butter' that's solid at room temperature. But shea literally melts on contact with the skin, to produce a deceptively light, spreading oil. The trees grow in 19 countries across the savannah zone of Africa, from Senegal in the west to Ethiopia in the east, where it has been a beauty staple for centuries, as well as a cooking oil. The West African shea (*V. paradoxa*) tends to be slightly thicker than the East African (*V. nilotica*), which is why you might find different types in skincare.

Shea is not a quick crop: the first plum-like fruit are produced when the tree is about 20 years old, it reaches maturity around 45, then goes on producing fruit for up to 200 years. I passionately believe that it's vital to buy shea butter – as with many crops, particularly those grown in developing countries – that's sustainably grown and fairly traded. One of my own research projects is with women's cooperatives in Uganda and southern Sudan, where the shea butter is harvested without either slave or child labour and a fair price is paid direct to the growers.

The abundance of fatty acids (linoleic, linolenic and arachadonic, sometimes collectively known as vitamin F) and high content of antioxidant vitamins A and E has made shea a useful ingredient in moisturisers and hair conditioners (and it sometimes can turn up in chocolates, too). It's quickly absorbed, non-irritant (so can be good for inflammatory skin problems such as rosacea) and doesn't clog pores.

A volume of research suggests that green tea may help to combat the mechanisms that play a role in initiating skin cancer

healthy cells, while ushering cancer cells to their deaths. Dr Hsu believes that using green tea extracts may help not only with wrinkles and sun damage, but psoriasis and rosacea too. As with other plant extracts, it's important to choose good-quality products that contain sufficient levels of green tea extracts to deliver these benefits.

Natural vitamin E
(d-alpha-tocopherol)

I could practically write a book just about this wonderful skin-friendly substance, mainly derived from vegetable oils, which was discovered in 1922. It wasn't until 1962, however, that its role as an antioxidant, which could delay skin ageing, was proposed. Used in cosmetics, natural vitamin E (more than twice as powerful as the synthetic version) helps to defend the skin from the damaging effects of ultraviolet light, to optimise moisture levels and improve appearance, and to delay skin ageing by fighting free radicals. One of the main ways it works is by protecting the phospholipids (fatty acids) in cell membranes, which form the 'cement' of the skin barrier and are major targets of attack by free radicals. It also improves wound healing.

Although it's used mainly in cosmetics, doctors are increasingly interested in it too. Research shows that vitamin E can reduce acute and chronic skin damage from UV radiation. Scientists from the Department of Dermatology at the University of California wrote in a medical journal: 'regular application of skin care products containing antioxidants may be of the utmost benefit in efficiently

Green tea
(*Camellia sinensis*)

Renowned as a health-giving and disease-fighting drink for at least 3,000 years (a reputation that's supported by current scientific research), green tea is increasingly found in skincare. This is due to its powerful antioxidant activity, which combats the effects of free radical damage and also acts to quell inflammation. Scientists believe that the antioxidant polyphenol compounds derived from this fragrant shrub help to prevent sun damage and thus the signs of premature ageing. Research suggests that it helps to combat the mechanisms that play a role in initiating skin cancer, so green tea extracts are mostly used in anti-ageing and suncare products. Dr Stephen Hsu, a cell biologist at the Medical College of Georgia, Augusta, helped determine that polyphenols in green tea safeguard preparing our skin against exogenous [external] oxidative stressors occurring during daily life', adding that sunscreens could also benefit from a combination with antioxidants. Vitamin E actually exists in the stratum corneum but, while some antioxidants can be synthesised by humans, this 'essential nutrient' must be obtained from our food (fresh vegetables, vegetable oils, cereals and nuts) and by topical delivery, according to leading researcher Jens J Thiele of Boston University Medical Center. Since the majority of people fail to meet the current recommendations for vitamin E intake, there is a big argument for using well-formulated moisturisers to protect your skin and also taking a supplement of natural-source vitamin E.

Hyaluronic acid
or sodium hyaluronate

HA, as it's known, is one of the newer wonder ingredients touted by the beauty industry. The thing is, it might be just that. HA is natural to the body, where it carries out many crucial roles, notably lubricating our joints. It also acts a shock absorber and, together with collagen and elastin, forms the scaffolding of the skin, which gives tone and 'bounce'. Because of its remarkable ability to attract and bind water, HA – also an antioxidant – has been nicknamed 'nature's sponge' and one of its functions is to hydrate the all-important collagen fibres.

The American Food and Drug Administration has approved the use of animal- and non-animal-derived HA as an injectable dermal filler, which testifies to its safety. Research has shown that topical application of HA helps wound-healing and can reduce scarring. Some research suggests that, unlike most compounds, topical HA can penetrate the epidermis to hydrate skin tissue and plump up wrinkles, as well as helping to give a more velvety texture. It is definitely an important ingredient in skincare and, I predict, will become more so.

The main source of HA is rooster combs, but, for people who prefer not to go down the animal route, it is also available in non-animal form. (Soy beans are used as the source of HA in Liz Earle skincare formulations, which are all cruelty-free.)

Watch this fruit!

In Kenya, my smaller children laugh at a tree called *Kigelia africana*, known as the sausage tree, because of the shape of the huge, cylindrical fruit, which weigh between 5–10kg and dangle like salamis in a deli. Kigelia has a long history as a medicinal plant, applied topically. The dried and powdered fruit is used in Africa to clear the skin and for eczema, acne, ulcers and infections caused by wounds, insect or snake bites. In southern Africa, according to Prof Peter Houghton of King's College, London, it has a considerable reputation for being effective against solar keratoses, which may develop into skin cancer. Women in Africa rub an ointment made from the fruit pulp onto their breasts to tighten and firm the skin, as well as enlarging their bosom (or so they believe). The extract from these unusual fruits does seem to have skin-tightening properties and it's one to watch out for in future skin firmers. I've now discovered that certain active compounds have been found in Kigelia, including one called kigelinone; this comes under the group scientifically called napthoquinones, some of which are being researched for their anti-inflammatory action on the skin. Other extracts from this amazing fruit have shown antibacterial activity, which probably accounts for its anti-acne properties.

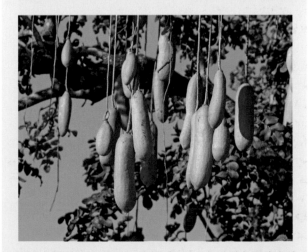

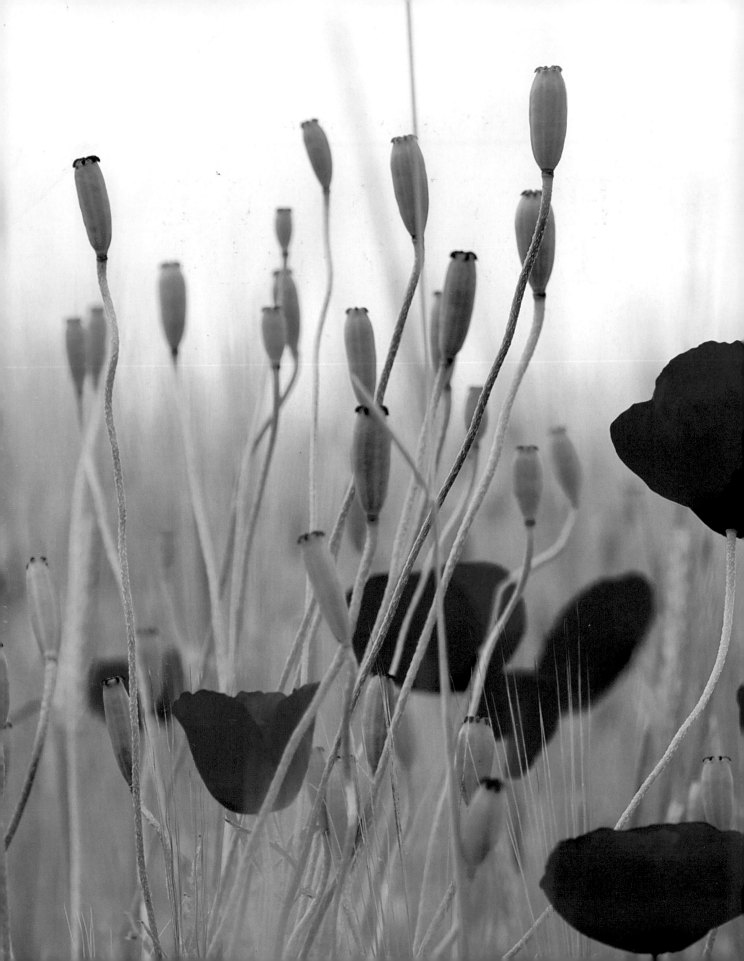

Chapter Three

HOW TO HAVE LOVELY SKIN

Our skin's needs change over the decades
and in this chapter I share some of my secrets
for each age and stage of your life, from teens
to seventies. There are even a few
pages for men...

How to have lovely skin … in your teens

Teenage years are a time of change – and this is especially true for your skin. Here's how to give skin the best start.

What's happening

The cells of the skin are being produced at an optimum rate now, so it is renewing itself about every 28 days, and your complexion should be peachy, plump and bright. Collagen and elastin in the dermis are functioning perfectly, making skin toned and resilient. But hormonal changes mean those in their teens (and even earlier ages, these days) may have problems with blackheads, whiteheads and acne because hormones called androgens increase the production of sebum or oil from the sebaceous glands. Dead skin cells stick to the sebum, blocking the oil ducts – the sebum's getaway route – resulting in blackheads (or whiteheads, which are basically the same, except that they have not been exposed to air and dirt). Behind these blocked pores, the acne bacteria grow rapidly in the sebaceous glands, triggering inflammation and redness. You may also find that your skin tends to be shiny because fluctuating hormones affect sebum production.

TLC for your skin

The basic products you need are a cleanser, toner and daytime moisturiser, plus sun protection if you're outside or on holiday. Let your skin breathe at night, rather than loading it with a night cream, although you might stroke in a few drops of a lightweight oil, as I shall explain. Bodywise, you shouldn't need much, except perhaps an occasional body scrub (useful for keeping skin smooth, so you don't get patches if you're self tanning) and a body lotion if your skin is dry.

Thorough cleansing is essential – even after the wildest night out, when you just want to flop into bed – but don't strip your skin of its natural moisturising oils. A minute's massage with a creamy cleanser (not soap: it won't shift oil or oil-based make-up effectively) wiped off with a clean muslin cloth or flannel, wrung out in warm water, is all you need. This will also keep your pillow clean – important, because debris-laden pillows can trigger spotty skin. Cleanse your face first thing in the morning, too, to wipe away sebum produced overnight.

Toners are useful just after cleansing, to remove any residue and brighten and refresh the face. You could use aloe vera juice, which is healing and soothing, for spot-prone, inflamed skin (see page 128): choose a brand that is sold fresh in the refrigerated section and store in the fridge to help preserve its vitamins and enzymes. For oilier skin (not dry) mix three parts rose water with one part witch hazel.

In the daytime, follow with a moisturiser based on lightweight but emollient plant oils, such as a mix of coconut and palm oils (look for coco-caprylate/caprate on labels). This mix has very good spreading power, yet a non-greasy – almost dry – feel. Also look for products with added antioxidant, such as beta-carotene and vitamin E.

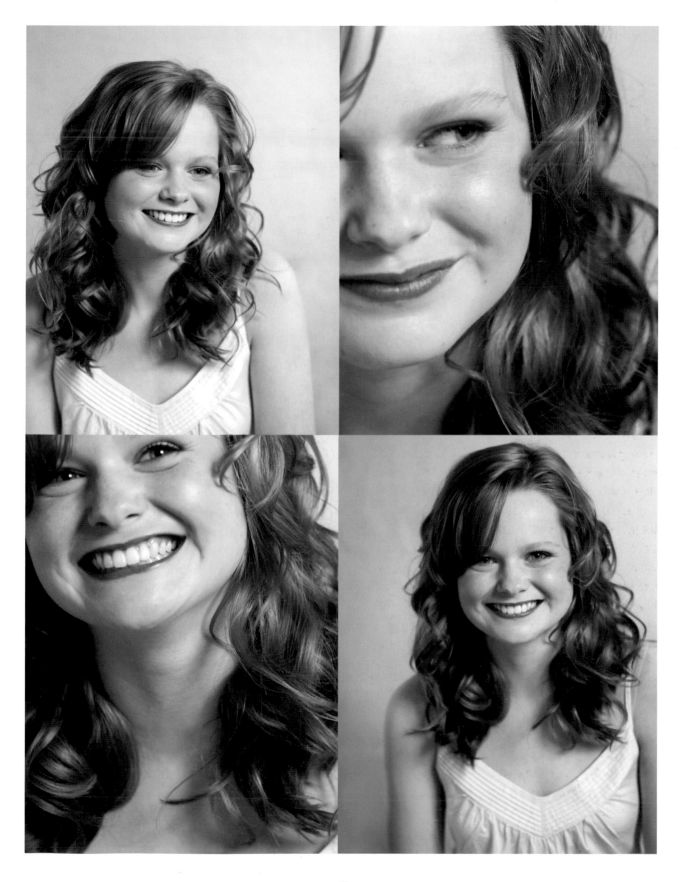

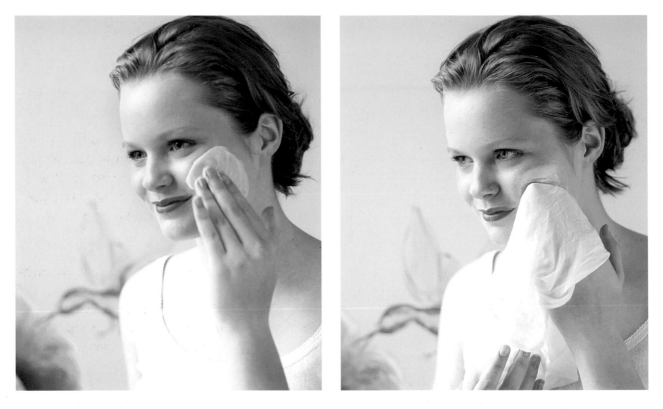

A cream-based cleanser, removed with a muslin cloth wrung out in warm water, is the best way to cleanse the skin and a good habit to start early

Although most teens aspire to look tanned, a much safer option is to self-tan. Keep skin protected when in the sun, apply a mineral-based sunscreen, with a blend of titanium and zinc oxide filters for broad-spectrum protection against UV light, which suits even the most touchy skins.

If you're enviably spot-free, choose a simple range that you enjoy and stick with it – chopping and changing may provoke your skin. Learn to read ingredient labels: all products carry an INCI listing (ingredients), which will guide you through much of the jargon. Learn to read your skin, too: notice when it feels tight, taut or over-dry – usually due to over-stripping with harsh drying ingredients, such as benzoyl peroxide. Soap, even so-called 'mild' facial soaps, can also strip the skin, over-dry it or lead to sensitivity.

If you have oily skin, avoid ranges that claim to cut

Secret
Zap spots with milk of magnesia, lavender or tea tree essential oil dabbed on a cotton bud – or a tiny spot of toothpaste. All three dry sebum and are antiseptic.

oiliness and dry the skin: the skin may then produce more oil to compensate, setting up a vicious cycle. In fact, I don't believe in buying oil-free skincare for face or body: remember, our skin produces its own oil, so oil, as such, is not bad. I suggest using lightweight plant oils, such as apricot or peach kernel or passionflower seed oil. Massage in a few drops on your face at night to soften sebum so it can get out of the follicles and help balance your skin.

Choose formulations without mineral oil (*paraffinum liquidum*), as this can clog pores. This inevitably means going for a 'greener' or more natural option. Skincare ranges targeted at teens – often labelled 'non-acnegenic' – aren't necessarily best (there is no legal definition of 'non-acnegenic'). My advice is always to treat angry, inflamed skin with great care, using calming and soothing ingredients such as natural clays, manuka honey and propolis. A teaspoonful of a gentle herbal extract, such as calendula (marigold), chamomile or hypericum (St John's Wort) tincture, in a bowl of warm water makes a gentle face splash. Calendula ointment is very calming for sore, red skin: I especially like the Nelsons range, usually found in the homeopathy section of chemists and health stores.

Make sure your hands are washed before touching problem skin. Pustules can be encouraged to come to a head by applying a cloth wrung out in hot water to the affected area. Very gently remove any pus with the cloth; be sure to wash it thoroughly after. A greasy fringe can trigger spots on the forehead, so keep hair pinned back and make sure skin and hair are kept scrupulously clean.

If you have oily, spot-prone skin on your back or chest, cleanse the area thoroughly every day with a gentle body wash. A towelling backstrap is useful for reaching upper backs, but do wash it and your bath towel frequently – daily, if you have acne. Applying a clay-based, deep-cleansing face mask to the affected area once or twice a week can also help: do your face at the same time.

Making up

My teenage daughter Lily loves Benefit's High Beam, a pearly pink liquid which you dot on cheeks and brow bone for a healthy glow. It's actually multi-age: she gave me a pot for Christmas to stop me stealing hers!

✳ The best eyelash curlers are Shu Uemura: they are expensive, but a good investment – and a great present.

✳ To subdue shine, try Origins Zero Oil, which blots shine to an instant matt finish without drying, or Body Shop Matte It Face & Lips, which suits all skin types.

✳ If you have a breakout, dot on a cream concealer with a (very clean) eyeliner brush, pinpointing the red epicentre – then cover with a fine brushing of translucent powder.

✳ Blotting papers are useful for on-the-spot shine treatments (try MAC or, in the UK, Barbara Daly for Tesco), or simply peel apart a paper tissue.

Secret

Secret

Lip balms or sticks made with mineral oil or petroleum jelly don't re-moisturise, they simply sit on the surface. More natural ingredients, such as plant oils and purified lanolin are the best choice for keeping lips soft and comfortable.

✳ Mineral make-up, which contains skin-healing zinc oxide, sits better on the skin than thick foundation and gives some sun protection. Prescriptives' All Skin Mineral Foundation SPF15 (a powder) claims to be concealer, base and finisher in one, and is good for hiding teenage blemishes without clogging.

Nutritional needs (also see page 187)

✳ If you have dry skin, take an essential fatty acid supplement with omega-3 and GLA (gamma-linolenic acid). It may take 2–3 months before you see results so don't give up too soon.

✳ If you have spots, consider vitamin A; also zinc with copper to help heal acne and prevent scarring.

✳ I also recommend colloidal silver, which you apply directly to spots, or mix a few drops with your daily moisturiser. This naturopathic remedy can really help to keep skin clear as it de-activates the enzymes that cause bacteria to multiply.

Treat

Treat

Ask for vouchers for a professional make-up lesson – take a friend for fun! It will save you lots of money on unwanted products and give you confidence. You can also book in for (usually free) make-up sessions with brands at a department store: if you can't decide which brand, stroll round and note the consultants you like the look of, then sign up.

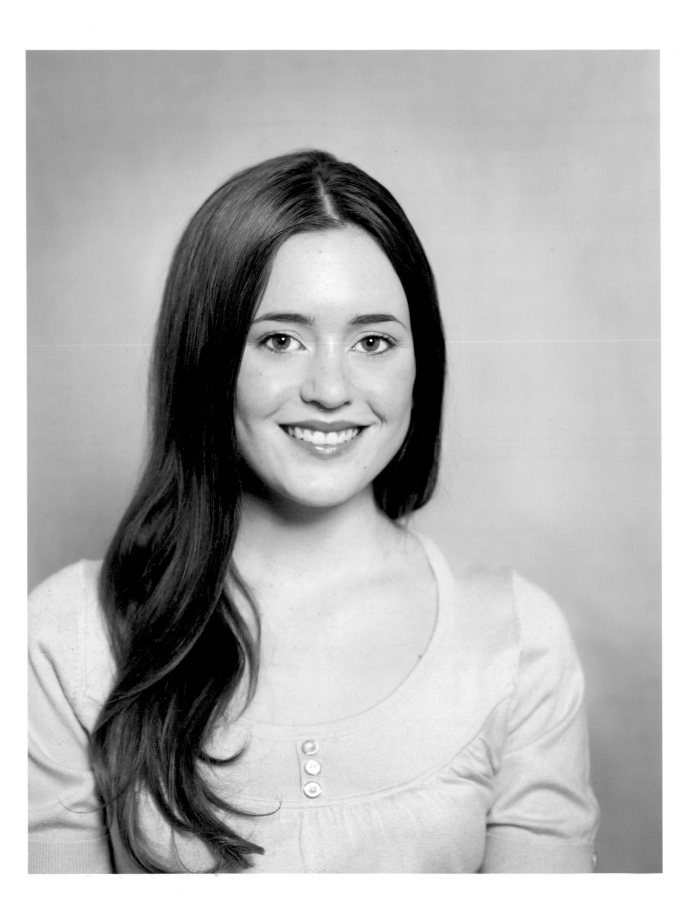

Lovely skin ...
in your twenties

Most hormonal changes should have taken place by now, so this is the perfect era to establish good skin habits.

What's happening

In my experience, skin should be settling down by now and behaving reasonably normally. However, those with relatively high oil production may still have spots and/or shiny skin, likewise blackheads and whiteheads (particularly if you live in a polluted environment).

Line-wise, your face should still be silky-smooth, although fair skin which hasn't been protected from the sun may show the beginnings of sun spots and crows' feet.

Those who drink too much or smoke may see the beginnings of broken blood vessels, early sags and bags, and a dull, unhealthy-looking, spotty complexion: remember – your skin is often a barometer of the way you live. Bodywise, you may still experience spotty breakouts on your back, or skin pimpling and rough patches on the backs of arms and legs.

TLC for your skin

The core products I suggest for your face are a cleanser, which you remove with a soft muslin cloth or flannel to exfoliate gently, an alcohol-free skin tonic, light daily moisturiser, slightly richer night cream, facial oil and mask. Look after your body with a scrub (to use every few days) and body lotion (for daily use), plus suncare for both face and body.

Whichever your skin type, start exfoliating very gently, just enough to remove the top, dead layer of skin cells on your face (and body, see below). In the mornings, buff it with a soft muslin cloth (or fine towelling flannel) wrung out in warm water. This is also a good way to remove any cleanser at night (in fact, the Liz Earle Cleanse & Polish Hot Cloth Cleanser was specifically formulated to use this way).

In the morning, follow with a sweep of alcohol-free skin tonic (or pure aloe vera gel) and a light dab of daily moisturiser. Useful ingredients in both skin tonics and moisturisers include antioxidants to protect against free-radical damage and essential fatty acids to help keep skin smooth. I also like echinacea for its skin-toning properties and calendula or chamomile for their mildly anti-inflammatory, skin calming benefits.

Those with combination skin are often given complicated advice. I treat all skin types in the same way for cleansing and toning; then for combination (and oily) skin I suggest light day moisturisers and night products, plus specific mattifiers that will blot excess sebum, such as clay-based treatment masks and blemish treatments on the oily areas.

Oily and combination skins can use the same daytime moisturiser at night, to nurture all skin types. However, normal or dry skins may lap up a slightly richer, more hydrating night cream with ingredients such as avocado, borage seed or evening primrose seed oils. I avoid creams containing mineral oil (*paraffinum liquidum*) as it can clog pores, encouraging acne.

Another skin secret is to massage in a facial oil last thing at night, to cherish all skin types, as plant oils help balance and regulate the skin. Dry or normal skin responds well to avocado, argan and rosehip oils. Lightweight plants oils such as peach, apricot kernel and rosehip suit oily or combination skin. Because such oils are similar to sebum, they help 'persuade' the skin not to produce an excess.

Avoid products that dry the skin (they often contain benzoyl peroxide) because they also strip it of oils: the skin's immediate response is to produce more oil so people then use more aggressive products. It's a vicious circle. Look for ranges with gentle purifiers such as witch hazel, rosemary and eucalyptus. (Also see pages 128–129 for more detailed advice on acne.)

Anyone still suffering with acne on their face and/or body should see their doctor and request a referral to a dermatologist. If you have breakouts round the time of your period, consider herbs such as chasteberry (*Agnus castus*). For skin scarred from acne, chicken pox or surgery, a daily massage with rosehip seed oil really helps, but the older the scar, the longer it will take to fade. You should see some improvement after three to four weeks' regular use, though. Add a few drops to your usual moisturiser or blend your own facial oil, using one tablespoonful of base oil, such as apricot kernel, to a teaspoonful of rosehip seed oil.

Nourish your face and neck with a weekly mask and select one according to your skin type: intensive moisturising for drier and normal skins, deep-cleansing for oily/combination.

Use body scrubs to gently buff away patches of dingy skin. Dry skin body brushing is useful too (see page 92).

Please don't forget to use suncare on your face and body – and hands! Imagine your face as a shrivelled-up old prune in a few decades and take protective action now. If you are on the contraceptive pill, you may find you get brown stains on your upper face, cheeks or upper lip. These pigmented patches occur because the hormones in the pill, as with pregnancy, increase the production of melanin, the tanning pigment. If you sunbathe too, you get a double effect, according to dermatologist Dr Nicholas Lowe. You can't completely prevent this condition, known medically as melasma or chloasma, but you can lessen the effect by using a sunscreen at all times (look for four-to-five-star SPF15-20) – even on cloudy days – and staying out of the sun whenever possible. UVA can pass through glass, so apply sunscreen even when you are in the car, or behind a window.

If you smoke, stop now for your skin's sake, if nothing else: apart from the mustardy-coloured teeth, facial lines, bags and saggy skin, you'll get a yellowish skin tinge.

Treat

Skincare is for sharing and a girl's night in is fun and wonderfully therapeutic if you're a bit stressed. Everyone brings two or three of their favourite beauty treats and swaps tips and treatments with a giggle and a gossip (and fresh juices or a glass or two of antioxidant-rich red wine…). It's a good way to try something new without costing too much as well. P.S. it's a lovely family thing to do too, with all generations from teens to granny, via mothers, aunts and cousins.

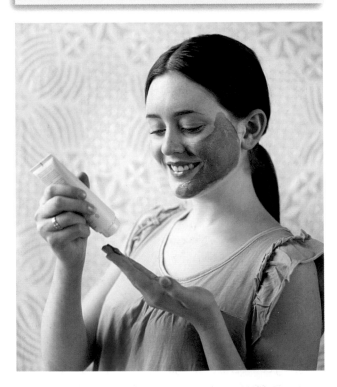

Clay-based masks help draw impurities from enlarged or open pores and temporarily (some say permanently) improve their appearance

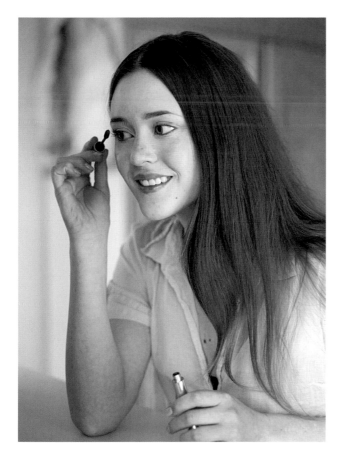

mixing a tiny amount of Yves St Laurent Radiant Touch (Touche Éclat) in your palm – to warm it – with the same quantity of a liquid/cream foundation: Chanel Teint Innocence is a wonderful light fluid base for any skin. Ruby and Millie's Concealer Duo, which you apply after a base, is brilliant too. Whatever you choose, dot it on very lightly with your ring finger, building up thin layers to cover.

● A 'pop' or dot of pure colour, blended well into the fleshiest part of cheeks gives an instant lift and glow when you smile. NARS blusher in Desire – a super-bright fuchsia which tones down on the skin – looks amazing.

● MAC Face and Body Make-up is an excellent, lightweight liquid foundation. It comes in an array of shades: I use shade C2 on my face and upper chest, and on bare legs for summer evenings out as it gives a healthy, lightly tanned gleam and subtly hides thread veins and patchy bits.

Tip
Breathe out when you apply powder to avoid particles going up the nose!

Making up

For shiny faces, use a water-based foundation and carry shine-absorbing facial blotters. Translucent powder blots shine and also sets foundation, giving it more staying power. I like Laura Mercier's Translucent Powder, which isn't cheap but lasts for ages.

● My London-based make-up artist and friend Kerry September swears by Guerlain's Teint de Matte foundation. MAC. also makes excellent oil-free bases, including Studio Fix Fluid SPF15 and Select SPF15, plus a water-based tinted moisturiser, Select Tint SPF15.

● If you have spots, leave your face bare of make-up for a couple of days so it can heal: draw attention to your eyes and lips instead, with mascara and a little shimmer on the eye lids, plus a gorgeous lip gloss.

● When you really must conceal spots or other blemishes – including dark circles – remember the aim is to make the concealer look like a second skin, NOT a mask. Bobbi Brown Foundation Sticks may do everything you need, or try

Nutritional needs (also see page 187)

● A good vitamin and mineral formula is a daily skincare insurance policy and tops you up with skin-saving nutrients, especially at times when you eat less well. I started taking Advanced Antioxidant Formula or VM75 by Solgar Vitamins in my twenties and have never stopped. If you're not already taking a product with GLA (gamma linolenic acid) and Omega-3 essential fatty acids, add one now to encourage skin smoothness. Keep in the fridge to ensure freshness.

● If you have spots, consider Vitamin A (this has also helped PCOS sufferers with intractable acne).

Secret
Keep skin clear and smooth by sipping 6–8 big glasses of still water every day (between meals). Sipping little and often rehydrates better than knocking back a couple of large glasses at once.

Lovely skin …
in your thirties

It's during this era that your skin will start to show visible signs of ageing – more or less, depending on how you treat it.

What's happening

If you've protected your skin really well from the sun and other climatic extremes, it may still be bright and blooming. But that's the exception: most of us notice some dullness as cell turnover slows and the stratum corneum (the surface 'horny layer') retains dead cells.

There's almost certainly some environmental damage in the epidermis; it may be invisible but reckless sunbathers will probably have sun spots and possibly even small, scaly, pre-cancerous skin lesions: do consult your doctor if you notice any suspicious signs. Those on very low-fat diets – and, of course, smokers – may notice dullness, dryness and the start of significant lines.

With collagen and elastin fibres not working as efficiently, your dermis is likely to be losing some of its bounceback. Stress can affect collagen formation so, if you're under pressure, look for ways to relax: more on this in Chapter 9.

Creasing of the skin from repeated muscle activity (eg. frowning) can begin to show now, with the start of a central trown furrow, lines across your forehead and crow's feet. Look at your mother and grandmother to see how particular areas age, then take specific action.

Bodywise, things won't be as youthful and taut, and you may notice drier, even rougher skin.

TLC for your skin

This is the time to really boost hydration outside – and from the inside, so sip at least eight large glasses of pure, still water daily. The basic products you need for your face are cleanser, alcohol-free toner, day moisturiser, night cream and/or oil, eye product, exfoliator and mask.

For your body, I suggest a rich top-to-toe body cream, as well as an all-over body exfoliator/scrub to use in the shower once or twice a week – and, of course, sun protection for every bit of exposed skin.

Cleansing and moisturising remain the most important activities. Choose a cream-based, detergent-free facial cleanser to work in harmony with the skin's slightly acidic pH balance (the 'acid mantle'). I never use anything that foams on my face as it's too drying, even for oilier skins – and can trigger the production of even more sebum. A cream cleanser also works well as an eye make-up remover, even on stubborn waterproof mascara. I always advise using a soft cotton muslin cloth to remove cleanser and whisk off dead grey skin cells.

Follow cleanser with a sweep of skin tonic/toner sprinkled on a soft (beware rough, scratchy varieties) cotton wool pad. Toner not only feels refreshing but can temporarily minimise enlarged pores. Choose an alcohol-

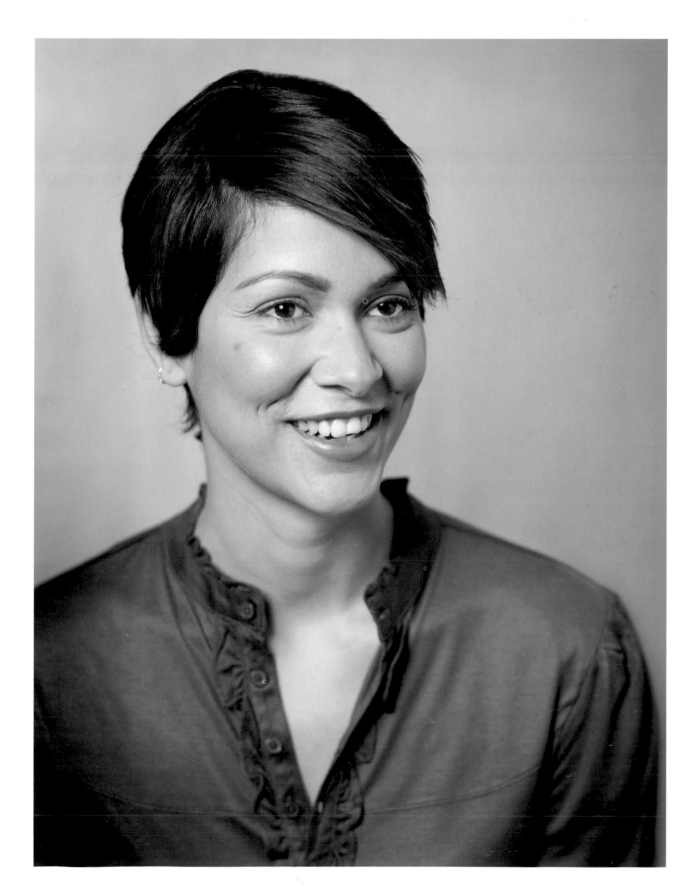

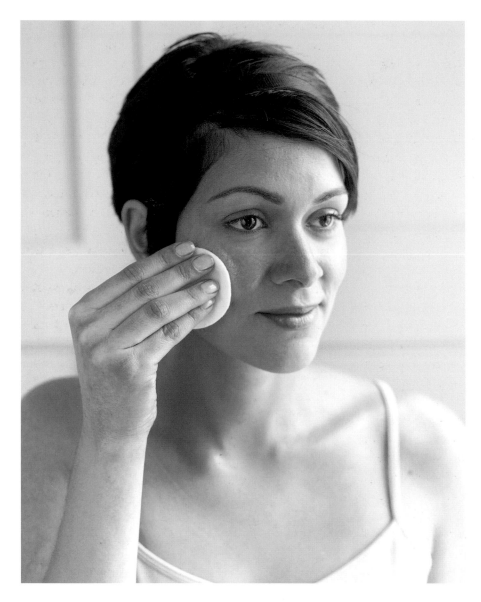

Humectant ingredients are also beneficial, including glycerin and hyaluronic acid (sodium hyaluronate).

If you have combination skin with an oily T-zone, choose a lighter moisturiser, formulated for normal/combination skin. Even if your skin is oily, it's still worth using – sparingly; the merest trace of a very lightweight cream with antioxidants and essential fatty acids will do. It's really important if you live or work in an urban environment to help shield your skin from airborne pollutants that trigger free-radical damage.

While sun protection is key to prevent premature skin ageing as well as skin cancers, I don't believe in using an SPF in a moisturiser. The amount of protection is small and the SPF mostly wears off by lunchtime. My advice is to buy a separate facial protector, ideally SPF20,

free formulation that won't overly dry or irritate: a little is OK, but you don't want to see 'alcohol denat' near the top of the ingredients.

Select your moisturiser according to your skin type, making sure it's based on plant oils, not pore-clogging mineral oil (*paraffinum liquidum*). Dry skins tend to feel taut after washing and need a rich cream packed with skin emollients, such as avocado, wheatgerm and rosehip seed oil together with borage or evening primrose seed oils, which are full of essential fatty acids to moisturise deeply.

with mineral sun screens (a blend of titanium and zinc oxide) and apply a fine layer over your moisturiser when going outdoors. If you wear make-up, the mineral ingredients should provide a protective veil equivalent to about SPF10–20.

For small 'sun' or 'age' spots on your face, massage in a little rosehip oil mixed with the contents of a vitamin E capsule every night; during the day always cover with a concealer or face-specific sun block. If the backs of your hands have sun spots, try a hand cream rich in vitamin E

Safety at work

Many of us at this age work in offices, which can take its toll – and not just in mental stress. Resting a grubby phone handset on your face can provoke breakouts in previously clear skin. Clean the handset with an alcohol-based cleanser or wipe. Get your eyes tested if you frown at your computer screen: the right specs can make a big difference to forehead furrows (and stop headaches, too). Air conditioning can dehydrate the skin, so you may need a richer facial moisturiser on working days.

(natural source – d-alpha tocopherol – is more effective than synthetic) and use your facial SPF on your hands, too.

Get into the habit of using an eye cream, as it will help to keep the finer skin around your eyes smooth: use daily, for best results. You don't need lots of eye products: a good formulation should deliver several benefits. Look for one that contains natural skin plumpers such as GLA, antioxidants and richer plant oils, such as borage seed, rosehip seed, cranberry seed and/or avocado. It should preferably contain a mineral sunscreen, such as titanium and zinc oxide – so you need to apply it in the morning, rather than at night. Some under-eye creams also contain light-reflecting particles which can help banish the appearance of dark circles and shadows by 'bouncing' the light away from the skin. Wearing big Jackie O-style sunglasses with 100 per cent UVA/UVB protection and wide arms will help prevent lines round your eyes.

You can double up by using your daily moisturiser as a night cream, as long as it doesn't contain a sunscreen. But if your skin is very dry, you may want to switch to a slightly heavier – richer – night cream. The skin cells do more of their repair work whilst we sleep, so this is the best time for the cream to sink into the upper levels of the epidermis and moisturise. All skin types will reap rewards from a nightly application of facial oil: even oilier skins benefit from their gentle skin-balancing properties. Look for blends based on pure plant oils (not mineral oil – *paraffinum liquidum*):

lightweight facial oils include hazelnut, passionflower, peach and apricot kernel. Lightly massage into your face and neck, last thing; rub any excess into your cuticles and nails.

Giving your face a once or twice weekly exfoliation and mask is time well spent. Gentle facial exfoliators (make sure there's nothing scratchy in the product, such as jagged particles of nut kernels) pep up the skin by giving it an extra buffing and are ideal to use before applying a treatment mask. Choose a mask specifically for your skin type, such as a rehydrating mask for parched skins, or a clay-based one to draw impurities from spottier complexions (these also help absorb excess sebum). Take both exfoliator and mask down on to the neck and upper chest for best results.

Exfoliators, also known as scrubs, are brilliant body buffers and one of the fastest ways to improve the overall look and feel of your skin. Keep a tube of your favourite handy to rub into damp skin, especially on hips, thighs and

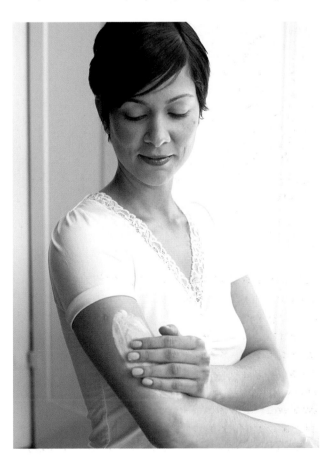

the backs of arms. Particles of olive kernels and ground pumice are great for body buffing. Safety note: avoid glass jars, which can smash in the shower.

Apply lots of body cream daily, from chin to toes, as soon as you have towelled dry after a bath or shower – it absorbs more easily into warm skin. Choose products with nourishing plant oils, such as shea butter, rather than mineral oils, as these sit on the surface, often feeling tacky, and don't rehydrate deeply.

Now is a good time to think about bust perk-ups, especially if you have a generous bosom or have been pregnant and breastfeeding. If you can't face a daily hosing with cold water (the results are guaranteed by beauty editors), you might want to include a specific product. Nothing short of the surgeon's knife will keep the bust as pert as a teenager's, but there are useful, non-surgical options. With regular use, specific skin-tightening bust gels and serums have been shown to tighten slackened skin – although don't expect a miracle. That said, good formulations can certainly improve skin hydration and should help overall tone and elasticity. Useful skin-toning ingredients include *kigelia africana* (sausage tree extract), quince and mangosteen – all proven skin firmers. Bust treatments are also a useful way to encourage you into regular checking for breast lumps, too.

Even if you are watching your weight, please don't go on a fat-free diet: it's more important than ever to make sure you get enough of the 'good' omega-3 fats, vital for your skin and the rest of your body – and your brain. If you are cutting back on fats, add in a daily supplement with a combination of omega-3 and omega-6; the calories are negligible but the benefits to your skin and the rest of your body, including your brain, are significant. You'll find more on this later in chapter 7.

From 30 onwards is the peak age of onset for rosacea, if you are affected by this inflammatory condition, which causes redness, pimples and prominent tiny blood vessels. Turn to pages 130–131 for specific advice.

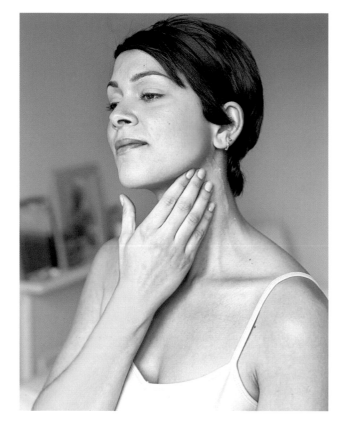

Skin on our necks can start to look crepey in our thirties, so extend your facial skincare down the neck to the upper chest

Ions

In a natural, clean, outdoor environment, the balance of negative (good) and positive (bad) ions in the air is about equal. But in enclosed indoor spaces, particularly with computer monitors and other office equipment, the negative ions are claimed to be depleted, leading to tiredness, headaches, allergies and, possibly, to less good skin. There is some science to suggest that negative ions can boost collagen and improve the functioning of skin cell membrane, also helping the delivery of oxygen to cells and tissue. As well as getting out of the office into clean air as much as possible, consider investing in an ioniser: but choose one from a reputable company.

Eye crayons are a versatile addition to every make-up bag. Test before buying to make sure they have a soft, creamy consistency that won't drag delicate skin

Making up

✳ If your skin is looking a little tired and in need of an instant 'lift', try Chanel's Base Lumière, an illuminating primer that you can use under foundation or even on its own to give skin a natural luminosity: it looks as if you've had several nights' excellent sleep.

✳ As a foundation, I suggest Giorgio Armani Luminous Silk Foundation; it's oil-free, leaving your face matt but not dry. (Beauty editors have raved about it for years.) L'Oréal's oil-free formulations are also good.

✳ Eye pencils add instant colour and are brilliant for travelling. Deep, soft grey works well on all colourings: I like RMK Deep Grey, and there are plenty of good, budget-priced pencils by brands such as Max Factor and Bourjois.

✳ For make-up on the run, my instant kit consists of an eye pencil, plus a Stila Convertible Colour cream blush in 'petunia' for cheeks and lips, which I top with a Stila 'Mango' lip gloss.

✳ To create a fabulous pout, dab a touch of white-ish highlighter, such as Benefit's High Beam (or any pale pearly shade from your eyeshadow compact), in the cupid's bow of your upper lip, to emphasise the lip line.

✳ If you've never had your eyebrows professionally shaped, book in now! For some, it's the equivalent of a non-surgical facelift. If you're doing it at home, don't overpluck them in the middle. Hold a pencil vertically from the inner corners of your eyes to your brows and pluck hairs within that area only. Generally, pluck hairs from underneath brows only, although if the arch is very sharp and your face narrow, just even out the top a tad to widen your face and give a graceful curve. Soothe skin afterwards with a sweep of alcohol-free skin toner.

Nutritional needs (also see page 187)

✳ Taking a high absorption form of vitamin C with minerals will help maintain the collagen network. I take Emergen-C sachets when travelling.

✳ Continue taking a multivitamin/mineral and an essential fatty acid supplement.

✳ A natural source vitamin E supplement is useful to help guard against premature skin ageing by minimising free-radical cell damage.

Treat

Spoil yourself with a professional facial: choose a brand you really like and seek out experienced local facialists. For real pampering, recruit someone to pick you up afterwards… so you can totally switch off and relax.

Lovely skin ... in your forties

It is said that life begins at forty and, all being well, you will be in the prime of your life. But skin changes fast during this decade and good skincare can make a real difference both now and for the future.

What's happening to your skin

This is my decade, as I write this book, so believe me – I know! This is the stage where all the processes governing your skin – both face and body – start to slow down. But while you wouldn't expect to have the peachiness of youth at fortysomething, you can still have lovely skin.

This is where women with oily skin come into their own: for the rest, the natural reduction in sebum (oil) production brings drier skin and the potential of lines. My skin is drier than the Sahara at the best of times so I have to work really hard on this one. But I still manage to keep it relatively smooth with plant oils, without resorting to injections of facial fillers or freezers.

Generally, at this stage, women don't experience a loss of subcutaneous fat – unless it's in your genes – but you may notice less plump lips. Cell turnover is slowing down too, so the top layer of dead skin cells (stratum corneum, or horny layer) tends to become thicker and less bright.

The big change is likely to be the breakdown of collagen, with a loss of elasticity. Bluntly, your skin is likely to become slacker, particularly around the jawline. Your body skin may show signs of drooping, too, with a threat of the dreaded flabby upper arms.

Menopausal changes typically start around 44, often bringing stress, poor sleep (due to night sweats) and spotty outbreaks in some women. Declining levels of oestrogen, which keeps skin moist, supple and soft, contribute to skin dryness and lack of suppleness. Hair also tends to become drier and more brittle: the growth generally slows, though in some this self-corrects after your final period. Eyes may become drier too.

Sun damage in the form of brown spots and patches may appear now, though less so if you've been vigilant with your suncare.

TLC for your face and body

The key products I suggest for your face are a creamy cleanser, gentle facial scrub, non-drying skin toner, day moisturiser, night cream and oil or serum, face mask, plus a multi-purpose balm for lips, cuticles and the rest! For the body, a body scrub, rich body cream, hand and foot creams, plus a dry skin brush.

Moisturise – just as much as you can! Face, neck and cleavage (very important!) in the morning and top to toe at night or after bathing. Make it part of your routine and you will be amazed by the results... good creams sink in fast.

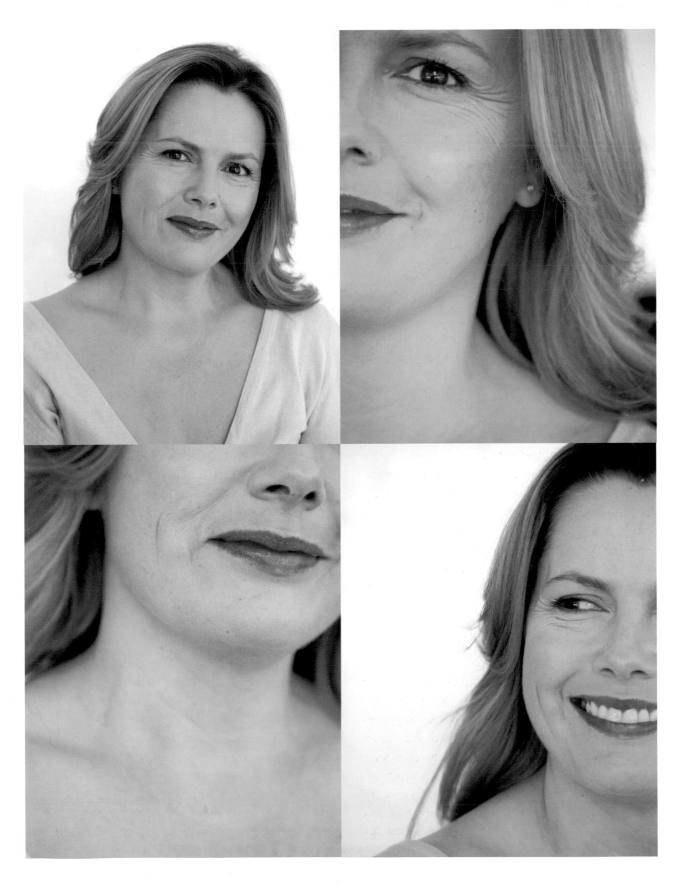

Look for products that promise believably youthful skin benefits. My favourite ingredients are plant-based because these bring so many benefits to ageing skin, particularly antioxidants and essential fatty acids. I love avocado oil, rosehip seed, borage seed and passionflower seed oils, as well as the magical argan oil (see page 27). Obviously I use Liz Earle skincare, but I use the richer formulations now I am in my forties. There is evidence that botanicals can be just as effective as high-tech 'anti-ageing' synthetic compounds, sometimes more so. The surveys on Liz Earle Superskin Moisturiser (which I use now) scored an incredible 98 per cent for skin plumping among the 60 testers after four weeks' home use.

Plant oils also make the best base for body moisturisers because they are so quickly absorbed into the upper epidermis. If a body cream contains mineral oil, it feels tacky after applying, although the skin beneath still feels dry.

To help the stratum corneum on the surface of skin release its thick coating of dead skin cells, gently exfoliate at least once a day with a soft face cloth. Use a more intensive treatment once a week or so. But do choose a type with smooth, round beads – often labelled 'spherical' – that buff and don't scratch, unlike crushed shells, pumice, salt or sugar grains, which are angular. (Natural brands tend to use jojoba beads, high-tech ones polyethylene.)

Facial exfoliation shouldn't stop at the chin: gently buffing neck and upper chest helps keep ageing skin softer and smoother. For the body, I switch to a grittier formulation, with slightly larger polishing particles, such as ground pumice, sugar or salt. French actress Carole Bouquet told me one of her top body beauty secrets was to mix a handful of fine sea salt with a handful of olive oil to use in the shower. It really leaves the skin gleaming (just be careful not to slip on a wet surface). Dry skin body brushing can help even out the bumpiest-looking skin, and also combat cellulite by giving blood and lymph a boost (see page 92).

Bath oils are another wonderful way to literally soak up the goodness of these moisturising marvels. A dessertspoonful of almond, apricot or peach kernel oil softens even the most parched skin and is especially useful during winter months.

And don't forget your hands – the more hand cream, the better. If nails are flaking, apply oils direct to your nails and also take them as a supplement – suggestions on pages 100–1.

Do give your feet some TLC as well – see my advice on page 102 and try to visit a qualified chiropodist every six months, quarterly if you have foot problems. Well-kept feet not only look good in their own right, the comfort factor will show in your face.

Moisten dry eyes with a spray such as Clarymist, which doesn't disturb make-up (spray at 20cm) and has been clinically proven to help treat dry eye syndrome. To help reduce eye puffiness, I fill a basin with cold water, plus ice cubes if they're handy, and splash my eyes ten or so times, then pat dry with a soft towel. I can see the puffiness diminish within minutes.

Skin sensitivity is often an issue now, so look for products with fewer ingredients and be selective. Even the chemical components of natural essential oils, such as citral and linalool, can trigger allergies. If anything makes your skin itch or tingle uncomfortably, stop using and check

Apply oil directly to your nails to prevent flaking and to encourage stronger nail growth

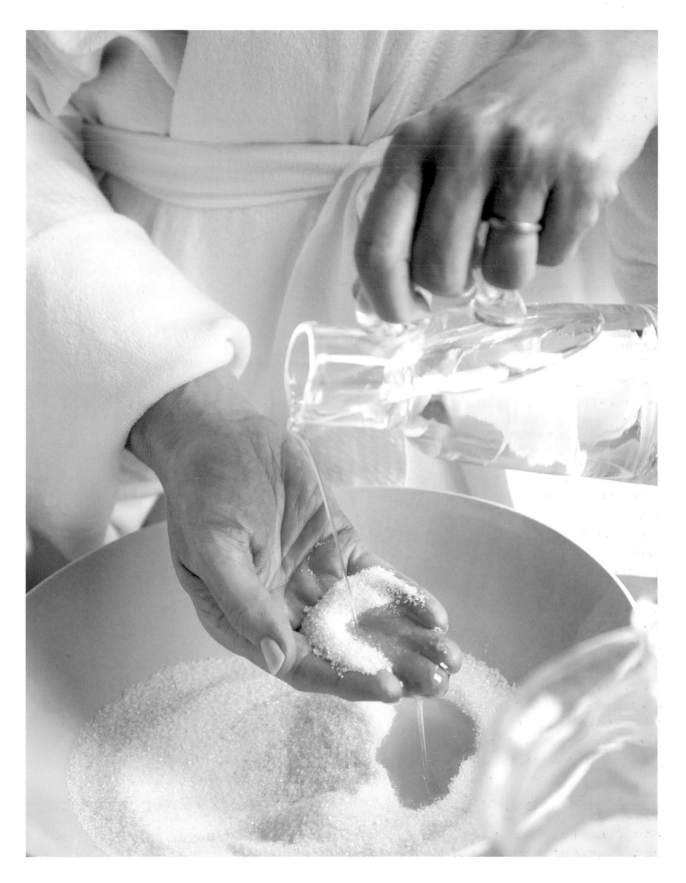

the label for a potential culprit. (There's a useful A-Z of ingredients in the 'Green Pages' on the Beauty Bible website, www.beautybible.com) If your sensitivities become severe, ask your doctor to refer you for skin sensitivity patch testing.

If thread veins and broken blood vessels are a problem, see a dermatologist or specialist vein clinic. The only effective method of removal I have found is sclerotherapy – injecting tiny amounts of saline to seal off the leaking capillaries. If you're prone to redness, avoid extremes of temperature such as saunas, hot steam baths, or freezing plunge pools.

Stress affects collagen production (which also impacts on your bones, in terms of osteoporosis – see Nutritional Needs, below) as does lack of cell-repairing sleep, so find ways to relax, such as yoga, meditation or prayer – and balance these with exercise you enjoy, which can be as simple as a walk in the fresh air.

Hot flushes

With these, keeping your make-up on can be a challenge. Here are some tips from women (and a man!) who know.

❋ Opt for tinted moisturiser or a very light foundation. US-based make-up artist Craig Beaglehole recommends Giorgio Armani Luminous Silk Foundation – one of my favourites – or MAC Face and Body water-based foundation on its own (I use C2), or mixed in with your moisturiser in your palm.

❋ To get foundation looking natural, Craig suggests putting a dab in your palm, mixing it with your finger tips, then pressing on to your face. 'Massage it in to create a veil of foundation that blends into your moisturiser and skin,' he says. 'This way, if you do have a hot flush, your base won't go streaky.'

❋ Craig suggests a light dusting of featherweight powder to set foundation or tinted moisturiser, 'so if you have a hot flush, you can just let your face dry and your make-up is still there.' Take your base and a pressed powder compact in your bag for a quick freshen-up, he advises. Stila Sheer

Colour Face Powder is a great option, or Clinique Gentle Light Pressed Powder.

❋ For more hold, add blusher after powder. Craig's favourite gel blusher is Stila Convertible Color (try lilium or peony) and, for a powder formulation, Nars Powder Blush.

❋ Craig suggests using a waterproof mascara, such as L'Oréal Architect Waterproof Mascara, which 'simply does not move', according to Craig.

Hot sweats don't seem to touch lips, so invest in your favourite, most flattering lipstick, gloss and matching lipliner. Always have facial blotters – paper tissues will do, says Craig – plus a small atomiser filled with spring water and a drop each of essential oils of juniper, clary sage and geranium. Shake well and spray on your face and neck to cool you down. (Do not use on rosacea.) Some skin tonics also come in a spray or spritzer version – look for those rich in aloe vera for on-the-spot cooling and refreshment.

Making up

✳ My favourite foundation in my forties is Estée Lauder's Futurist Age-Resisting Make-up. I love the radiant, dewy finish it gives; it comes in two formulae, for dry or normal/combi skin. I use the shade Blonde 13. I also rate the Dermablend range of extra-strength concealers, originally developed to cover birthmarks and scarring. These are especially useful on areas of changing pigmentation.

✳ Make-up artist Bobbi Brown has a silky Shimmer Blush that looks fresh and natural but really lasts. I also like Nars The Multiple stick for cheeks and eyes: the naughtily named Orgasm shade gives skin a fabulous glow.

✳ For eyelids, I like pale beige and biscuit tones (Bobbi Brown has a great palette), plus a thin trace of gel eyeliner (MAC or Bobbi Brown). Apply the thin line close to your lashes with a thin, stiff brush.

✳ To help give definition and a flattering contour under the cheekbones, I use Laura Mercier Mineral Powder in Warm Bronze, applied gently with a large blusher brush.

✳ Barbara Daly advises using a lipliner pencil to create a crisp outline which looks youthful, but it must be in a natural colour – a dark line round paler lips is very ageing.

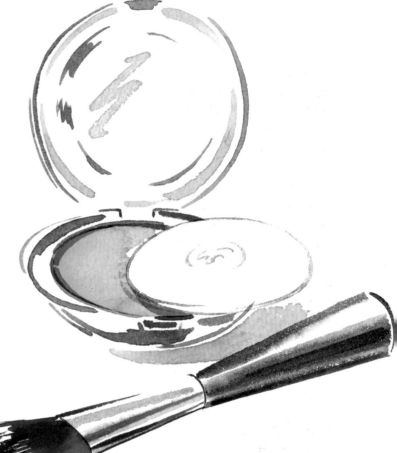

My weekend 'no make-up' kit is edited down to these few favourites:

✳ Stila Convertible Colour cream blusher in Petunia to give cheeks a healthy glow

✳ Bourjois Beige Rose 08 stroked across eyelids for subtle definition

✳ Lancôme Definicils Mascara in Black to lift and frame eyes (I have been using this for twenty years as it is simply the best).

✳ Dr Lipp Original Nipple Balm For Lips or Liz Earle Superbalm to smooth and shine lips
That's it!

Nutritional needs (also see page 187)

✳ Phyto-oestrogens help balance hormones and protect the skin against premature ageing. Ladies Choice contains small quantities of nine plant oestrogens, plus a heart protective compound. Friends who I have given this to say it is very good.

✳ Antioxidants including SOD (supraoxidedismutase) help protect the skin against free radical damage.

✳ Make sure of getting your beauty oils by taking a product with GLA (gamma-linolenic acid) and Omega-3 essential fatty acids.

✳ Calcium and magnesium supplements are crucial from now on, as bone degeneration may already be occurring.

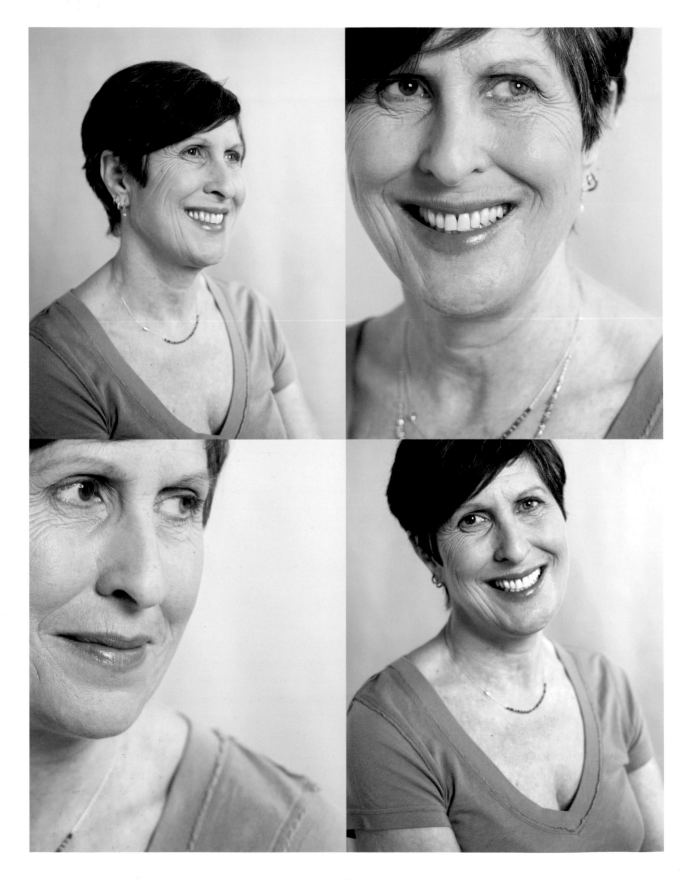

Lovely skin ...
in your fifties

Looking and feeling fabulous is the aim and there's lots here that can really help.

What's happening to your skin

The best thing about this decade is that everything starts to settle down, though you may have a bit of a bumpy start – the average age of a woman's last period is 51 and menopausal symptoms such as hot flushes may continue for a few months. By this point, oil production is really slowing down and most skins will be getting drier. The oilier-skinned among you will be at a big advantage now.

The breakdown of collagen and elastin, mainly due to declining oestrogen, means that the structure of the skin becomes looser and you may start to notice dewlaps. Also, the padding of fat over your cheekbones may start slipping, altering the contours of your face: this will be significant for skinnies – a good reason to consider putting on a few pounds. Fashion designer Carolina Herrera once told me that 'a woman of "a certain age" has to choose either her face or her backside'. Personally, I'd opt for plumping the face, as this is seen by rather more people.

Skin is also likely to be thinner and more fragile, primarily due to the decrease in collagen in the dermis. This makes it more sensitive, particularly to UV radiation and pollutants – but even to skincare that has never upset your complexion before. Confusingly, although melanin production declines overall – skin literally fades with age – it's more likely to be overproduced sporadically, resulting in pigmented 'age' spots or patches. The most common trigger is sunlight, so these tend to appear on exposed areas, principally your face and backs of your hands.

TLC for your skin

My mantra here is give your skin a helping hand, with extra protection, nourishment and hydration. As sebum (oil) production declines and the skin is also more fragile, it's more important than ever to support the skin barrier by applying oils.

The products I suggest you use daily for your facial skin are a cleanser, toner, daytime moisturiser, night cream and an oil, a day and night eye cream or serum, with a gentle exfoliator and mask for weekly use. Some experts suggest a neck cream but my experience is that taking your moisturiser and night cream from bosom to hairline works well, even for dry skins.

Always use a cream-based cleanser, never soap, as it is too alkaline for drier skins. Avoid anything that foams on the face, as that usually means it contains a detergent, most likely sodium lauryl sulphate (see page 13).

Exfoliation is very useful, as it helps to shift the top dead layer of skin cells, leading to visibly fresher, brighter and – crucially – smoother-looking skin. The key is to keep it gentle! Don't be tempted by dermabrasion or pot-scouring type buffing pads. You only need a soft cotton cloth to gently dislodge the dead grey skin cells. Use this with your cleanser morning and evening, and once a week give your skin a boost with a specific exfoliating treatment. Choose one with tiny round beads that gently buff the skin (natural jojoba beads or synthetic polyethylene ones), not jagged particles of ground pumice or nut kernels, as these can cause microscopic scratches and irritation.

Follow your weekly facial buff with a generous layer of a moisturising and firming facial mask. Exfoliate first, so the active ingredients of the mask can penetrate the upper layers of the epidermis. Choose an intensive nourishing treatment that's specially formulated to remoisturise: ingredients I like include St John's wort or avocado oil, and GLA (from borage or evening primrose seed oils).

Even dry skin benefits from using a toner, removing any last residue of cleanser and brightening the skin, but avoid any product containing alcohol, which will overdry your complexion. Many formulations include remoisturising ingredients, such as aloe vera and vitamin E. Skin toners can also help to calm flushed faces: look for products with anti-inflammatory ingredients such as cucumber, chamomile and calendula.

When choosing a day moisturiser, opt for a formula containing plant oils such as avocado, apricot or peach kernel. Make sure it also includes antioxidant vitamins or extracts: look for vitamin E, beta-carotene, green tea, grapeseed and pomegranate extracts.

If you spend time outdoors, layer a sunscreen on top of your moisturiser. Choose one made with broad-spectrum mineral sun filters (titanium dioxide or zinc oxide), rather than synthetic chemicals (such as cinnamates or benzophenones), which can trigger sensitivity.

At bedtime, give your skin a generous layer of goodness to feast on overnight. Massage in a few drops of facial oil first – choose a blend of pure plant oils such as rosehip, argan, evening primrose or borage seed – then turbo-charge with night cream. At this age, you need to switch to a richer product – the thicker the better; just make sure it has no mineral oil in the formula, as this is occlusive and won't let other ingredients sink into the epidermis.

It's also the right time to add a good eye cream or serum, specifically formulated to help fill out lines around the eyes. I'm a fan of hyaluronic acid (often called sodium hyaluronate), a naturally moisturising skin sugar, which

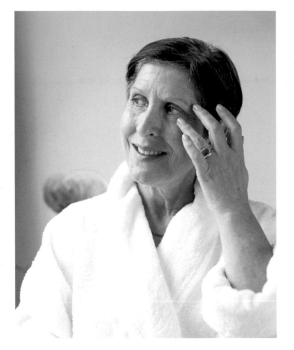

Use a good eye cream/serum to fill out lines around the eyes

really helps plump out facial lines. I also like to see high levels of essential fatty acids, including GLA and omega-3s. Use these products along any crevices, to subtly fill them. It's a myth that eye creams clog the skin: you can use them anywhere.

Bodywise, a good moisturiser is essential. Make sure this is based on pure plant oils and doesn't contain mineral oils – they are less efficient and may clog pores. Treat yourself to a body cream, as this has a higher lipid content than lotions, and will keep skin softer for longer. Be lavish from chin to toe, after every bath or shower to help rehydrate the skin, rubbing a little extra into parched areas such as elbows, knees and heels. Look for products containing moisturising and nourishing plant butters such as cocoa and shea butter. Dry skin brushing will improve the condition of skin immeasurably and help to prevent cellulite (see pages 92 and 96).

Hands and feet will welcome as much daily TLC as your face. Hands give away your age at a glance – just look at those of any Botoxed beauty over the age of 50. So make sure your hand cream contains plenty of antioxidants – vitamin E is especially useful to help fade pigmentation spots, though it will take time – and always put on sun protection: easiest to rub on a dot of your face product. In general, rub a little of whatever you're putting on your face on the back of your hands. And whenever you apply a mask to your face, treat your hands too. Slipping on a pair of gloves is a great hand-saver: use rubber gloves for indoor chores, gardening gloves outdoors.

Facial massage will help increase blood circulation to the face (see page 90). Some experts say the extreme movements of facial exercise can slacken the skin over time. However, I do think a few specific moves are useful to help keep the underlying facial muscles toned and tauter. I try to do two sets of the following mini-exercises twice daily, after brushing my teeth.

1. Push your chin out and lift your bottom lip over the top one, hold for a count of five, release, then repeat ten times.
2. Pull the corners of your mouth downwards in a fiercely exaggerated grimace, stretching and tightening the muscles that run down the neck and into the collarbones. Hold and repeat as above.

It's also said that dancers and yoga fans never need a facelift because the movements keep their jaws and neck defined and smooth, as with the rest of the body.

Making up

✳ In general go for softer shades. Swap black mascara for dark brown, use a softer, more natural lip shade – in sheer rather than matt – and the same with blusher.
✳ A favourite base for this stage is Chanel's Teint Innocence, as it is slightly richer and more covering than most, but with a sheer, natural finish on the skin. Skin brighteners perk up dull skin, helping to give it a little extra glow. (Try Prescriptives' Vibrant Vitamin Infuser for Dull, Stressed Skin or Guerlain's Midnight Star.)
✳ Women with good skin who like a lighter look may prefer a tinted moisturiser to even out skin tone (good ones are Crème de la Mer and Revlon), plus concealer or foundation

only where it's really needed. Dust on translucent golden powder for evenings.
✳ Eyebrows may well become thinner and paler during this decade; opt for a light taupey shade of eyebrow pencil, rather than anything dark or with red in it.
✳ For thinning eyelashes, try supplementing with Eylure's individual lashes (the shortest are the most natural looking). They are excellent for filling out sparse patches. I just apply two or three 'sets' to the outer corners of my upper lashes. I have also tried the semi-permanent individual lash extensions, which are quite expensive, but worked very well (though not for as long as expected). They are a useful option for holidays, camping or travelling – or if you lose your lashes due to medication.

Nutritional needs (also see page 187)

✳ Carry on with Ladies Choice, beauty oils and antioxidants.
✳ Calcium and magnesium supplements are crucial from now on, as bone degradation may already be occurring.
✳ Add in hyaluronic acid to help lubricate skin and joints.

Simple yoga-style stretches can help retain skin tone

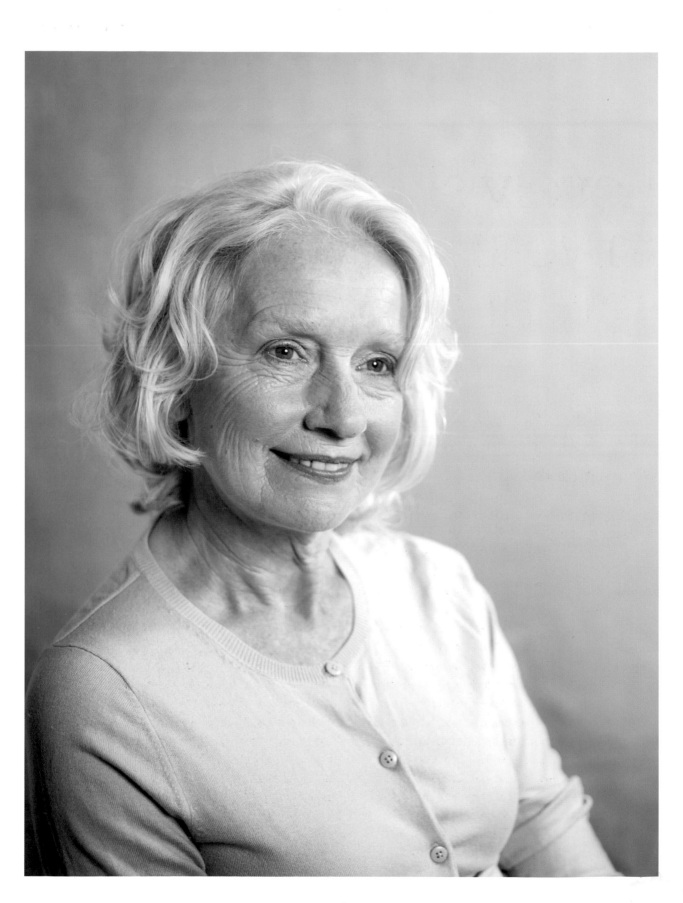

Lovely skin ...
in your sixties,
seventies and beyond

The good news is that it is never too late to make a difference to your skin – even in later years, visible improvements are possible.

What's happening

From now on, there's unlikely to be anything new as – at last – your skin stops being subject to the vagaries of hormones. What's more, the incidence of sensitive skin appears to fall with age and your face can even benefit from the ageing process: if you had a plump round face, you may find you have a more defined bone structure and the winged cheekbones you always longed for.

The downside is that the skin barrier declines as we get older, so more water gets out (TEWL or trans-epidermal water loss), increasing the problem of skin dryness. This is where plant oils really come into their own, as they provide the lipids necessary to strengthen the barrier. Your skin may also look paler, as the number of blood vessels reaching the dermis decreases: this can be helped greatly by exercising – and a bit of lipstick and blusher! Erratic overproduction of melanin may have contributed to dark circles under eyes, age spots and uneven colour.

In general, this is a time for intensive cherishing and daily maintenance: a little bit of TLC will reap radiance in your complexion. The motto for choosing products at this stage? Rich is good. No, I don't mean moneywise (you really don't need to spend a great deal) but with regard to ingredients – and also how much you put on. I counsel you to be lavish, from head to toe.

Remember, older women may not have the skin they had in their youth – but they won't have the spots either. And mature faces have a depth which can be immeasurably attractive. Your face is the sum of your life – so make sure it's as full of joy and humour as possible.

TLC for your skin

For your face and body, I suggest continuing with the skincare routine I outlined for women in their fifties (see pages 67–9). A valuable addition, however, is body oil, which will boost moisturisation in a way that a body cream alone can't quite achieve. Simply pour a dessertspoonful of almond, peach kernel or grapeseed oil into a saucer or the palm of your hand, add a scoop of body cream and mix. Apply this from chin to toe after bathing. (You can also add a little of one of the oils to your moisturiser or night cream.)

Incorporating massage techniques as you apply daily moisturiser and/or night products gives you a facial for free (see pages 176–7). Massage is particularly important during the winter, when the skin responds to the cold by closing down the small blood vessels in the dermis, which bring a glow to skin. This helps to prevent the body losing heat but leaves your skin looking dull, pale and somewhat lifeless. Be sure to stay warm, too: it will help keep your skin soft and lubricated by preventing excessive water loss.

If your eyes feel dry – which is normal, as mucus dries up – treat them to regular eye masks. Use cucumber slices, warm squeezed-out teabags (chamomile are particularly effective) or grated raw potato. Out and about, take soy-based drops, such as Clarymist.

Look after your teeth: gums slowly recede with time, but you don't want to add to the problem with gum disease, which can cause the lower half of the face to appear sunken. So floss twice a day, visit the dentist regularly and avoid sugar: if you use a sweetener, swap to xylitol, a delicious natural sugar that's proven to help strengthen teeth and bones.

Facial hair can be a problem; the easiest solution is to tweeze or wax away. All-over down (common on lower cheeks and chin) or moustaches also respond well to threading (see page 93).

When you go near the sun keep putting on the sunblock everywhere that's exposed. 'You can't be lazy with your skin,' says supermodel Carmen Dell'Orefice, still sensational in her late 70s. 'I practically go to bed with it on.'

Keep on eating as well as you possibly can; it can make a big difference. See my suggestions in Chapter 7.

Making up

● My observation from looking at glorious women in this age bracket is that the art is to use less make-up, but better. 'Colour is essential,' says US-based make-up artist

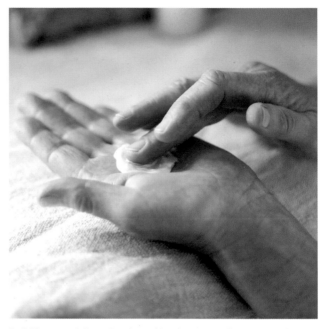

Enriching your daily moisturiser with a few drops of pure plant oil can make a big difference

Craig Beaglehole, 'because as you grow older, your skin and hair colour get lighter, so it's important to bring back that brightness with soft pretty colours and light textures – avoid hard lines and dark lips.' Aim for sheen, grooming and style, as well as femininity. 'Look like the most graceful and alluring lady in town,' as Craig puts it, 'with subtle make-up, well-kept nails, a great haircut and colour.'

● So what do you need, cosmetic-wise? The lightest base or tinted moisturiser, a radiant blush, a dusting of bronzing powder and a gorgeous lipstick in a soft but vibrant shade (rose, fuchsia, nutmeg or cinnamon, depending on your colouring) and a fabulous long-lash mascara. Remember that applying a double coat of mascara on the outside lashes is more becoming than loading on black eyeliner. Just stroke a whisper of colour on the lids – Nars make gorgeous sheer powder eyeshadows, which are long-wearing and crease-resistant.

● Do get your brows professionally shaped if you can (see page 59), and if you need to use a brow pencil, choose a light taupe rather than anything beetling!

Treat

A full body massage can smooth out aches and pains – and lines! Therapists invariably use oils which really improve your skin too. Find a local practitioner for the type of massage you like. There are all sorts, including aromatherapy, so spoil yourself – or ask for a voucher for your birthday or Christmas.

Nutritional needs (also see page 187)

● If you're not already taking a green plant food such as chlorella, consider starting now. Packed with good nutrients, chlorella (and its other algae relatives) are foods, rather than supplements. Chlorella is one of the most ancient water-grown organisms and, among other skin-nourishing properties, alkalinises the body – in other words, de-acidifies the gut. Regular users have noticed that their faces appear plumper and less elongated: this may, I'm told by a practitioner of traditional Chinese medicine, be down to the activity of two pairs of meridians which run down your face that are related to the health of the gut (see below). If the gut is alkaline, the meridians become relaxed, giving an effect which has been called 'a mini-facelift'.

● Additionally, carry on with Ladies Choice, Essential Oil Formula, GliSODin, hyaluronic acid and bone formula.

● If your digestion is dodgy (you suffer bloating, wind, etc), consider digestive enzymes. Such a supplement should also help with maintaining regularity. If you feel you need further colon cleansing, consider a detox (see page 158).

Facial meridians

I'm fascinated by the Chinese system of meridians so I asked Nadia Brydon, who is a qualified practitioner of Chinese herbal medicine and acupuncture, to explain a little more. She says: 'meridians are invisible energy channels just under the skin, first mapped by the Chinese over 2,000 years ago. They form an interlinking network of pathways along which the energy (Qi) flows. Acupuncturists insert needles at specific points along these meridians.'

According to Chinese medicine, Qi (pronounced 'chee') sustains all life and holds all the organs, glands, blood vessels, skin and body parts in place. If the Qi becomes weak – through ill health, say, or ageing – the body part or skin under which the meridian flows becomes loose and droops downwards. When the Qi flows strongly and freely through the meridians the body is considered to be balanced, healthy and 'uplifted'.

Each meridian is related to and named after an organ or function. There are 12 main pairs of meridians in the body that run either side of two central meridian lines. Several of these pairs of meridians run through the face, including the stomach meridian. This has the most visible effect, as it runs through the areas most noted for 'sagging' and 'drooping' as we get older (see illustration below).

Healthy foods help replenish the Qi lost through ageing, overwork, poor sleep, exhaustion, illness and poor diet. Jowls, double chins, sagging necks, breasts and tummy can all become more toned, plumped and smoothed out if we eat foods rich in Qi energy, including fresh fruit and vegetables and particularly chlorophyll-rich foods, such as green leafy vegetables and algaes (such as chlorella).

Exercise also helps activate the flow of blood and Qi in the body, reducing stagnation in the meridians and thus helping to 'lift up' the meridians and therefore the body as well as the mind.

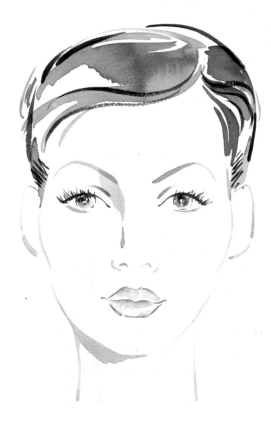

Lovely skin …
during pregnancy

Most of us bloom during pregnancy and a simple regime of cleansing and moisturising is often all you need. Here are a few optional extras that can also help with specific concerns.

What's happening to your skin

Pregnant women often have a soft, glowing skin, a radiance that's partly due to increased blood circulation during pregnancy, with more blood getting through to the tiny blood vessels in your skin, and also to the vastly increased levels of the reproductive hormone oestrogen, which keeps skin smooth, soft and supple.

But your skin can present you with some unpredictable dramas, too, also set off by the pregnancy hormones – oestrogen, progesterone and HCG (human chorionic gonadotrophin) – racing round your body. In addition, a growing foetus may deplete your nutrition levels, which can have a knock-on effect for skin. My teenage eczema returned when I was 28 and pregnant with my elder daughter Lily: it cleared up when I finished breastfeeding. Even if you've never had acne before, your skin may erupt during pregnancy. Or vice versa – women who've been spotty in the past find their skin actually clears up when they become pregnant.

The majority of women experience stretch marks; spider veins and varicose veins are common, and you may also notice pigmented patches (known as chloasma or melasma or 'the mask of pregnancy') on your face and body. Less common, but irritating, are itchy skin conditions (see page 76).

TLC for your skin

Hopefully, your complexion will be glowing, in which case you need the minimum of facial skin care. I suggest including a cleanser (be meticulous, if your skin is oilier than usual), alcohol-free toner, day moisturiser, a slightly richer night cream, plus a mask: stick to the suggestions for your age group in the previous pages. If your skin is misbehaving, try applying a facial oil blend each night to help re-balance it. Look for blends including avocado, argan and/or rosehip seed oils.

For your body it's a different story – more is better than minimum here. Avoid using soap, as it may be too drying: swap for a moisturising body wash formulated without sodium lauryl or laureth sulfate (SLS or SLES). Treat yourself to a tub of talcum powder in your favourite scent. This can help prevent skin chafing under your support bra and is useful dusted between your thighs in the summer.

Lavishing oils on your skin may help to prevent stretch marks (*striae gravidarum*). These look like pale-whitish-pinkish ribbons and turn up mostly on your tummy, breasts and thighs when the collagen and elastin are stretched beyond the point of no return. They seem to run in families and are more likely to affect older skin and fatter women. Women with darker skin are less likely to get them. Fortunately, they usually fade after the baby

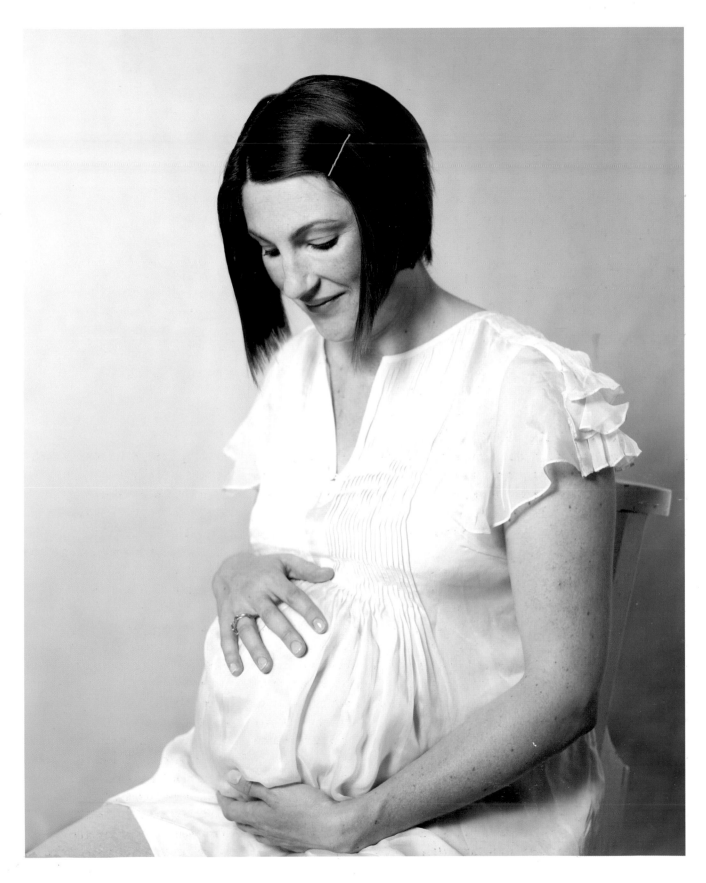

is born. All plant oils work well, but rosehip seed oil is the prime choice for helping to guard against permanent scarring. It's also worth piercing a capsule of natural-source vitamin E (d-alpha tocopherol) and adding this to the rosehip seed oil. If you have lasting marks, massage twice daily with a teaspoonful of this mixture.

Itchy skin conditions are another common problem. Some women suffer generalised itchy skin, which may be partly due to the stretching of the skin: keep your skin moisturised and try calamine lotion. One woman in 200 suffers from polymorphic eruption of pregnancy (PEP), a hives-like rash which begins on the stomach and spreads to the chest, neck, arms and legs during the last few months. It invariably disappears within two weeks after birth. Prurigo of pregnancy – itchy, raised, red or brown spots on the tummy, front of the legs or outer arms – affects one woman in 300, usually in the last three months. It may continue after the birth and/or in subsequent pregnancies. Discuss treatment with your doctor and eat plenty of oily fish (not tuna and swordfish, due to their high mercury content) and keep your skin well-moisturised. St John's Wort oil contains anti-inflammatory compounds that make it especially soothing, also calendula and chamomile lotions (from reputable   medical herbal or homeopathic companies, such as Nelson or Weleda.)

At bathtime, tie up a handful of oatmeal in a bag and attach it to a running tap to make the water silky and soothing.

Around 70 per cent of women experience the 'mask of pregnancy', darker patches of pigmentation around the face,

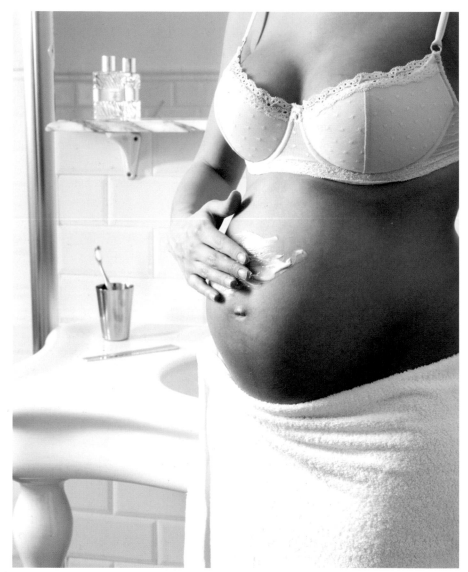

and sometimes body, due to oestrogen triggering more of the pigment melanin. Stay out of the sun, as this chloasma will worsen if your skin is exposed to UV rays; additionally, use a mineral-based sun protection factor 25.

Increased melanin production also means the skin around your nipples darkens; you might also notice a dark brown line (linea negra) from your navel to your pubic bone. As with chloasma, this pigmentation invariably fades within three months of giving birth.

Pregnancy hormones make the walls and valves in your veins more relaxed, and, with increased blood circulation, this may mean you get red or blue spider veins on your face, neck, chest, arms and legs. They usually only last as long as your pregnancy – so use concealer if you wish to camouflage them – but, again, are worse if you go in the sun. Dermablend make an excellent range of concealers, available worldwide.

For the same reasons, you could be plagued by varicose veins in your legs, thighs or groin. These swollen, itchy, sometimes painful veins run in families and are worse if you put on too much weight or stand a lot. They are likely to be troublesome in the last, heavy weeks of pregnancy, as blood tends to pool in your legs and lower body. When you sit or lie down, putting your feet up with ankles above chest height will help; massaging in an aloe-vera based gel will cool and refresh the skin. Sadly, concealer won't really help, but wearing good support tights will. Put them on before you stand up in the morning: I used to keep a clean pair ready by my bed. Avoid socks – or trousers – that restrict your circulation. Take gentle exercise, such as walking, swimming and general stretching (or yoga for pregnancy). If you have to stand or sit for long periods, make sure to walk around as much as you can. Avoid sitting with crossed legs.

In the last trimester, extra pillows placed under your side and knees in bed help support your lower back, so you tend to sleep better and that shows on your face.

Nutritional needs
(also see page 187)

✴ Doctors now agree that taking a supplement with omega-3 essential fatty acids is hugely beneficial for baby's health in the womb – as well as being good for you. These may be better than simply eating more oily fish, due to growing concerns over heavy metals in fish stocks. There is also some evidence that taking probiotics during pregnancy can help prevent eczema when the baby is born. (Remember, it's vital for the unborn baby that you have taken a supplement of folic acid if you're planning to get pregnant and during the first 12 weeks to help prevent neural tube defects).

Making up

✴ Most pregnant women have such a radiant glow they can ditch cosmetics except for a lip balm, tinted if you wish, and good mascara. I've been faithful to Lancôme Definicils mascara for over two decades. This classic is the only formulation that doesn't leave panda smudges under my eyes after a few hours but is easy to remove. Liz Earle Superbalm is a wonderfully versatile skin salve that did it all for me during pregnancy. I used it as a natural lip glosser, eyebrow smoother, to remove flaky skin and even as a frizz tamer for the dry ends of my hair.

✴ If your skin does go crazy at any point, US-based make-up artist Craig Beaglehole suggests Stila face concealers for blemishes, a cream-to-powder formulation in a cover-up stick which you pat on very lightly with a finger or brush. If you have high colour on cheeks, or for evening glamour, he recommends Stila Tinted Moisturiser or Prescriptives Traceless or a beautiful base such as Nars Balance foundation, which will even out skin tone but let your natural colour glow through. A tinted lip gloss and a whisper of colour on your eyelids, and you're good to go!

Treat

Have a pedicure so everyone helping to deliver the baby will see your pretty feet! Massaging the feet and lower legs is very helpful for blood circulation during pregnancy, so do treat yourself to more than one if you can. And more treats... If your budget permits, treat yourself to a facial: we store so much tension in our facial muscles, and lying on a facialist's bed, having your face and shoulders massaged, is so relaxing.

Super skin...
for men

When you've read this section, I suggest you might give the book to the man – or men – in your life, so he can read these simple guidelines to make his skin a little more gorgeous.

What's happening

Testosterone, the male hormone, dictates that, at puberty, along with a deep voice and big muscles, men develop thicker skin (20 to 30 per cent thicker than women's), facial hair – and usually rather more spots than the girls, because more hair follicles means more sebum. The anti-ageing upside is that, over a man's lifetime, the extra sebum provides an inbuilt moisturiser, while facial hair acts as a support structure, helping to prevent wrinkles. Men also have more collagen and elastin fibres and a tighter network of fatty tissue in the subcutaneous layer. (So basically they have an unfair advantage.)

Along with the facial fuzz comes problems, however: in a poll by the American Academy of Dermatology, 97 per cent of men shaved and 78 per cent of those reported skin problems as a result. The main ones were razor burn, ingrowing hairs, razor bumps, irritation and rashes.

Razor burn – characterised by rough, chapped patches, nicked skin and increased sensitivity – is caused by using a blunt razor or poor technique and usually disappears within a few days.

Ingrowing hairs can develop if the hair is cut too short, below the skin surface, or they may just never make it out of the skin. (This is most likely with curly hair, so men of African descent suffer the most.) Razor bumps (*pseudofolliculitis barbae*) form because the body treats an ingrown hair as an infection, causing swelling.

If the hair follicles become infected with *Staphylococcus aureus*, a bacterium which lives in the nose and gets into the follicles during shaving, it can lead to painful, itchy, red, pus-filled pimples – folliculitis, or 'barber's rash'. Mild cases respond to warm compresses of diluted witch hazel or white vinegar but, if the infection doesn't go away, do consult a doctor, who may prescribe antibiotic cream.

Long term, the main treatment is to shave correctly, as I explain below.

TLC for men's skin

Here's the mantra for men: wash, shave, moisturise. It really is that simple.

The best products for guys are a facial wash/cleanser, exfoliator, shaving cream and moisturiser.

For dry skins, choose a cream-based, non-foaming cleanser. Apply it all over skin before you put water on it, then remove with a muslin cloth or face flannel, soaked in hot water then squeezed out.

Oilier skins – ones that don't feel dry or taut after washing – can cope with a facial wash. Or even try a mild face and body wash, which you can use top to toe in the shower. But choose a gentle product that does not contain sodium lauryl or laureth sulfate (SLS or SLES), synthetic foaming detergents which can irritate and/or dry the skin.

Shaving exfoliates the beard area every day, but an exfoliant is useful around the nose and on the forehead.

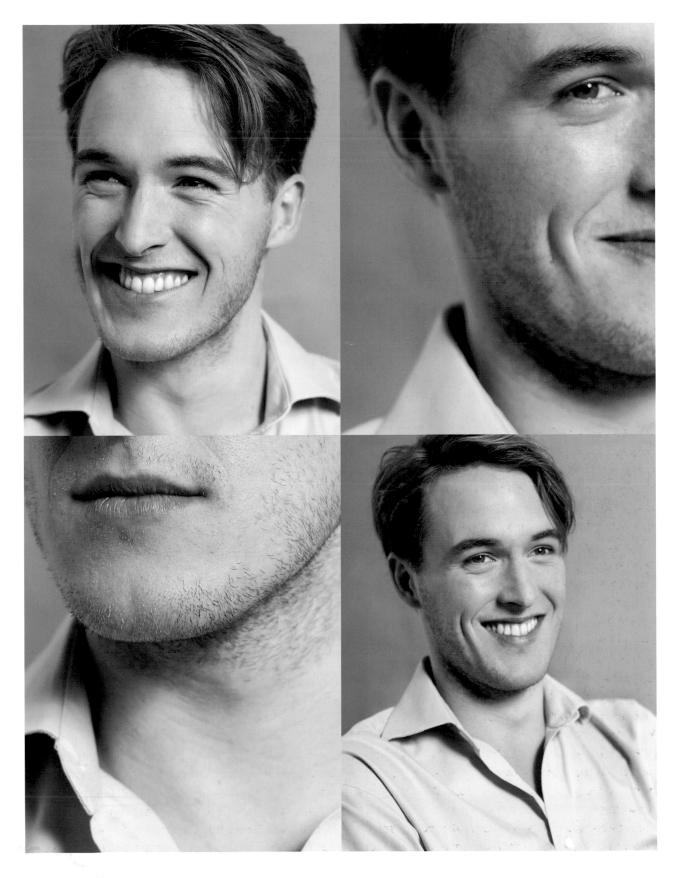

Use once or twice a week on the whole face; it will also unclog pores and discourage ingrowing hairs. Men's scrubs tend to be grittier than female versions to deal with tougher, thicker skin. Useful ingredients to look for include ground olive stones and pumice particles.

Watch out for shaving foams containing SLS or SLES, as they are so drying. I advise applying a non-foaming cream or gel in a thin layer, so you can see where the blade goes. My husband often steals my cleansing cream to shave with if his skin is feeling especially dry, and this is a good tip for those with sensitive skins.

As an aftershave moisturiser, a matt, lightweight lotion suits most men's skins more than a richer cream. Look for formulas that include anti-inflammatory botanicals, such as selfheal, aloe vera and calendula; the antioxidants vitamin E and beta-carotene help calm irritated skin, and GLA, an essential fatty acid, help improve moisture retention. Adding a few drops of antibacterial colloidal silver tincture to an after-shaving moisturiser can really help calm and purify the skin – keeping breakouts at bay too.

A couple of simple gizmos can make all the difference to overall grooming: I suggest a pair of slant-ended tweezers to pluck out stray, wiry brow hairs or nose hairs (take a deep breath and pluck on the out breath). Nasal hair trimmers are good and useful for hairy inner ears too: hold a hand mirror sideways to your bathroom mirror to check these.

Most chaps don't need much for their bodies, just a gentle body wash that can be used once or twice a day all over,

Acne

Acne tends to affect boys and men even more than girls. The linchpin is keeping your skin clean, eating well (low-sugar diet) and drinking plenty of water. The Ayurvedic herbal supplement Tejaswini contains twelve reputedly blood-purifying herbs used by Ayurvedic practitioners specifically to treat acne, pimples and cysts. It may be beneficial to take a product containing organic sulphur (MSM) plus essential fatty acids (especially omega-3 fish oils) to help keep skin healthy.

without causing irritation. If chafing is a problem anywhere, for instance the tops of thighs, shake on some unscented talcum powder (fragrance can be a skin irritant) or rice or corn starch powders. You can also dust this between the toes to help prevent fungal infections and keep feet smelling sweet.

Supplements (also see page 187)

However good your diet (and most men I know eat plenty, but not necessarily that well), international research over at least two decades shows that virtually everyone is deficient in one or more key nutrients, which are important for general health. So it makes sense to take a good multi-nutrient supplement. Pharmacist Shabir Daya recommends All Natural Perfectly Balance, which contains vitamins, minerals, enzymes, green foods and liver detoxifiers in a 'food state' for maximum absorption and utilisation by the body. I am also impressed by New Chapter Organics Every Man multi-formula, which I buy for my teenage son. My husband gets their Every Man II version for the over forties, with added Saw Palmetto, the herb linked to a healthy prostate, which may even help to prevent hair loss too.

Iron is as important for men as it is for women, but the concerns here are different (because men don't lose iron by having periods). During the early years (4–21), it is virtually impossible for men to accumulate an iron overload, as all the iron in the body is employed to produce red blood cells. In fact, boys may actually become iron deficient during growth spurts, ending up tired and sometimes suffering from concentration problems. Taking an appropriate multivitamin/ mineral supplement which contains iron should prevent this (eg, Junior-Vit by Health Aid). Alternatively, try a gentle preparation such as Spatone (which contains easily absorbed iron from a Welsh spa); take it in fruit juice, as the vitamin C content helps the body to absorb the iron. Once boys are fully grown men, they store iron and any excess can put a burden on the liver; it's also potentially linked with degenerative diseases of ageing, such as dementia, and possible mutation of cells, so iron is never advisable for cancer patients. Because iron has always been associated with strength and energy, men have tended to take more than they need. As a result, many iron supplements now carry cautions on the label.

If possible, bathe or shower before shaving, advises British grooming expert and TV presenter David Waters. 'Even better,' he says, 'eat breakfast first, as it warms up your facial muscles, which causes your beard hairs to lift up, making them easier to shave.'

How to shave perfectly

✳ Feel the direction in which your beard grows. This is the direction you should shave in.

✳ I recommend using a double- or triple-blade razor with a swivel head. To ensure it has a sharp edge, and minimise razor burn, change the blade every two weeks or so.

✳ For a quick shave, moisten your beard area by splashing your face with several handfuls of the hottest water you can stand comfortably.

✳ If you have a few extra minutes, soak a towelling flannel in very warm/hot water, wring it out and lay over your face for half a minute, pressing into all the contours. This can expand the hairs by over 30 per cent, making them easier to cut.

✳ Rub a small amount of shaving cream over your beard.

✳ Start shaving! Work in the direction your hair grows, using light slow strokes.

✳ Use your other hand to gently pull and stretch the skin, so you create a flat surface for your razor blade.

✳ While you're shaving, regularly rinse and tap the razor gently on the basin to remove hair and cream build-up.

✳ Smooth your hands over your face to check for any stray hairs; re-shave any missed areas.

✳ Splash your face several times with cold water to rinse and refresh the skin. Pat with a clean soft towel, leaving your skin slightly damp. Don't rub – it could cause irritation.

✳ Apply a moisturiser to soothe your face and lock in moisture to keep skin smooth.

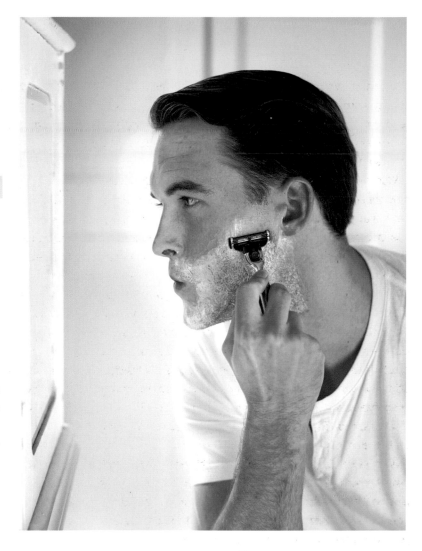

Always shave in the direction in which your beard grows. It may feel odd at first, but you'll get a closer shave and less irritation from razor drag

Treat

Invest in a magnifying mirror for your bathroom, either free-standing or a high-tech, wall-mounted version with a built-in light. It lets you see precisely where you are shaving and minimises the risk of nicks. For an occasional supertreat, have a professional wet shave at a traditional barbers.

Chapter Four

CARING FOR YOUR SKIN

A good skincare regime benefits every complexion, even the most sensitive – and it needn't be costly or complicated. Here's my advice for top-to-toe TLC, including an excellent rejuvenating facial, which is guaranteed to sweep away stress and make you feel and look better.

Caring for your skin from top to toe

The best skincare mantra is still the faithful 'cleanse, tone and moisturise'. But there's an addition: I believe exfoliating is the vital fourth step of all good skincare regimes.

If you're blessed with good genes you may have great skin, but good skincare can make healthy skin look even better – more radiant, softer and less lined. It can also help sort out (and prevent) problems such as breakouts and flakiness. Thorough cleansing is a vital part of our skincare process, especially if you wear make-up. Not only does it help to keep skin grime-free, it also prepares our face and neck to receive more nourishment from moisturisers and other useful creams, serums and oils.

I firmly believe a creamy cleanser is the best for all skin types. When my business partner Kim Buckland and I found that Cleanse & Polish worked for both our very different skins (Kim's oily and acne-prone, mine dry and sensitive), it was a revelation. As I have mentioned before, formulating Liz Earle skincare range was mostly down to enlightened self-interest: I couldn't find anything that really worked. Cleanse & Polish consistently comes top of consumer surveys (such as *The Beauty Bible* tried-and-tested trials), because it really does suit every kind of skin. It is packed with skin-calming and nourishing botanicals, but importantly doesn't contain any detergents or soap which upset the balance of the skin. We know, too, that very gently exfoliating the skin with a clean, damp muslin cloth lifts off dead skin cells, making skin immediately clearer and brighter and helping to speed skin cell renewal.

Toners, while not absolutely essential, are very useful to brighten up the skin immediately and visibly. Moisturisers, however, are a must. During my many years as a magazine beauty editor, finding a good moisturiser was the equivalent

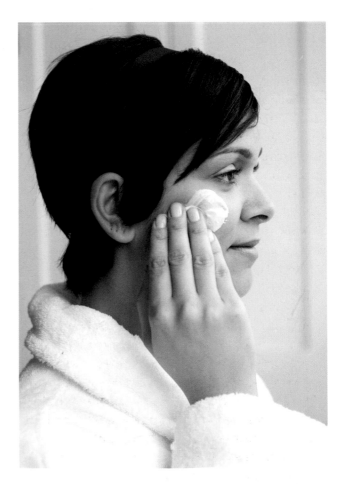

of the holy grail. An effective moisturiser slows down water loss through the skin, leaving it more dewy looking and plump. Also, unlike a cleanser, which is washed off, a moisturiser sits on the skin for many hours, soaking into the upper levels of the epidermis. This makes it an ideal medium to deliver topical benefits such as skin-plumping fatty acids, antioxidants to help repair free radical cell damage and soothing anti-inflammatory ingredients.

Absorption: what does and doesn't get through your skin

The subject of what gets through the skin and into the bloodstream via skincare absorption is a contentious one. Many beauty myths have arisen over the years and the media is fertile ground for promoting fearful scare stories. As a former journalist, later author and continual researcher, I have spent most of my working life investigating the more worrisome scare stories surrounding skincare. Some of the most common misconceptions I'm regularly asked about include the myth that up to 60 per cent (I've even seen 70 per cent claimed) of everything we put on our skin is absorbed into the body. This myth is a favourite of eco-warriors as it supports the rationale to use fewer 'chemicals' on the skin. Unfortunately, it simply is not true. Think about it: if we did actually absorb 60 per cent of what goes onto our skins the human race would be long gone, as our skin needs to be highly effective at keeping body fluids in and microscopic bacteria and viruses out, let alone much larger skincare molecules (we would also absorb huge quantities of water every time we went for a swim or took a bath…). Studies I have seen by the world's leading experts (professors and academics whose sole job it is to analyse skin permeability, not general dermatologists or other researchers) point to the fact that little can 'slip through' beyond the upper epidermis.

There are a few ingredients shown to penetrate the dermis though, notably synthetic sunscreens which are amongst the smallest molecules used in skincare. Studies looking at octyl salicylate (a synthetic sunscreen) show that after continual application for 48 hours the total amount absorbed is 1.58 per cent. Similar studies and data can be downloaded from www.rifm.org, the Research Institute for Fragrance Materials. Other academic organisations dedicated to studying skin permeability include The Skin Forum and they also have an interesting website www.skin-forum.eu.

The beauty world is rife with rumour and supposition, so it's well worth book-marking these credible resources to check whenever there's a skincare scare.

❋ www.the factsabout.co.uk
A newish site run by the Cosmetic Toiletry and Perfumery Association in the UK. Worth checking for a legally accurate view.

❋ www.senseaboutscience.org.uk
A UK charity for scientific information written by leading scientists.

❋ www.colipa.com
The European Cosmetic Toiletry and Perfumery Association website, especially useful for information on EU legislation and product labelling.

Some of the most common misconceptions I'm regularly asked about include the myth that up to 60 per cent (I've even seen 70 per cent claimed) of everything we put on our skin is absorbed into the body

How to get the best from your products

A few simple techniques will help you get the most from your investment.

Cleanse

Cleanse in the morning to remove overnight sebum production (to prevent spots) and in the evening to remove make-up and dirt. It is also good to cleanse when you get home at the end of the day, especially if you are a city dweller, to take off grime and pollution. (If you're staying in, let your skin go bare until you apply your moisturiser.)

Apply a small amount of creamy cleanser to the fingertips of one hand and dot on forehead, cheeks, chin and neck. Massage the cleanser into your skin in small circular movements – always work down the neck, and up from your jawline to your forehead, going outwards from the centre of the face. Work around the nostrils to help shift blackheads, especially if you're spot-prone.

If you are wearing foundation you may need to cleanse twice, first to remove all make-up and secondly to treat your skin.

Remove with a muslin cloth wrung out in warm water. Finish by patting the face with the cloth wrung out in cold water for a final refresh.

Tone

Sprinkle a generous amount of toner on a cotton-wool pad and gently smooth over your neck and face, working upward and outward from the centre. Keep your toner in the fridge – or pop it in for ten minutes before using – for maximum effect (it's especially cooling in hot weather).

Blot any excess with a tissue or dry muslin cloth to prevent it lying on your skin and making moisturiser less easy to apply.

Moisturise

If your moisturiser comes in a pot, load a cotton bud or plastic spatula with a blob about the size of a small coin – more, if your skin is dry. Alternatively, simply wash and dry your hands before dipping into the jar. Dot over your face, neck and décolleté before massaging in.

Moisturise morning and evening and follow with your eye cream, if using one. Even if you have oily skin, you should always moisturise. Just use a light lotion, applying the merest trace over your T-zone (forehead, nose and chin).

For extra-dry skin, I always apply moisturiser before adding a few drops of a hydrating face oil to further nourish. If your moisturiser contains mineral oil (*paraffinum liquidum*), you will need to use the face oil first as mineral oil leaves an occlusive film or barrier on the skin.

Eyes bright

To remove eye shadow, I like to use a non-oily liquid eye make-up remover on a cotton wool pad to sweep over eyelids. Dipping a cotton bud in remover is brilliant for taking off those last vestiges of mascara under your eyes – or whisking off errant smudges of eyeshadow during the daytime. I always use an eye cream that contains a protective mineral reflectant sunscreen; it also helps subtly conceal dark shadows and bags under the eyes, and saves on using an extra concealer.

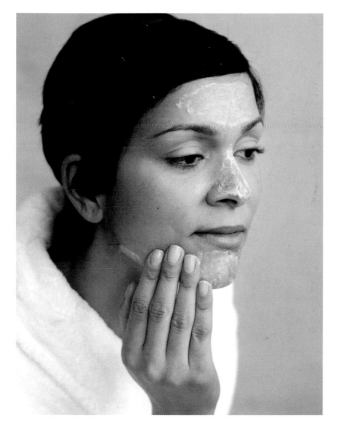

Exfoliate

Using a damp warm muslin cloth as part of your daily cleansing routine will give skin a gentle exfoliation.

Additionally, to give yourself the equivalent of a salon treatment at home, you can use a very gentle exfoliator once or twice a week. Look for ones containing spherical beads such as jojoba; avoid anything with jagged particles such as nut kernels. I don't believe in scouring pad-style dermabrasion: it's very harsh and may encourage inflammation, leading to free-radical cell damage and skin ageing. Little and often is a better approach.

Apply your exfoliator after cleansing. Mix an amount the size of a large coin with water (or cleanser if your skin is dry) in your palm. Gently massage this over your face, neck and décolleté, for one to three minutes, using the whole length of your fingers and working in little circles, out from the centre. Avoid your eye area.

To remove, first splash your face with water, then either use facial sponges from a chemist or a damp warm muslin cloth or face flannel. To remove any last traces, sprinkle toner on cotton-wool pads and sweep them over your face. Or remove by standing in the shower – it's quicker!

Tip

Exfoliating will double the effect of a face mask, so if you have time, follow up with an application of your favourite mask, leaving it on for 5–10 minutes. Your skin will feel velvety smooth afterwards.

Preservatives and skin sensitisers

The ingredients in everyday skincare have come under increasing scrutiny in recent years and there have been many scares regarding 'toxic toiletries' and similar sales-boosting headlines. We're often led to be afraid of 'chemicals', yet everything around us in the natural world, aloe to zucchini, is made up of chemicals. Anything claiming to be 'chemical-free' betrays its manufacturer's ignorance. Our bodies cannot distinguish between 'natural' chemicals and 'man-made' chemicals – it either utilises them as part of our metabolism or breaks them down for excretion. For example, ascorbic acid or Vitamin C have the same effect in the body whether obtained from citrus fruits or a supplement.

Another point of confusion relates to dosage. For example, propylene glycol can be a skin irritant, yet this applies solely to how much is used. In a skincare formula, it has the opposite function and is actually used for its skin softening and emollient properties, only being a hazard in its neat form (as with many essential oils). As an example, a glass or two of wine (around 13 per cent proof) is generally enjoyable, but a single glass of neat alcohol (around 95 per cent proof) will likely kill you before the day is out. Both are alcohol: it's a dose-related risk. It's worth putting ingredients into perspective when you study skincare labels, as small amounts of synthetics can actually be a power for good.

Other common scares surround preservatives and yet safe skincare needs to be just that, safe, – especially as we use it around our lips and eyes. This means using effective preservatives, especially in formulations containing water (listed as *Aqua* on the label) as these are most susceptible to contamination. Bugs love to grow and multiply in creamy emollients, especially in a nice warm, steamy bathroom environment. Recent studies by Professor Michael Cork and his dermatological team in Sheffield analysed moisturisers and found 44 per cent to be contaminated with bacteria, including 3 per cent containing the dangerous superbug MRSA. In one case, a small boy very nearly died from using bug-riddled moisturiser over open wounds on his skin. With deaths running in the many thousands each year from MRSA and similar 'superbugs,' the issue of properly preserved skincare has never been more important.

One family of preservatives are the parabens, also the subject of debate and controversy (it's been claimed they cause breast cancer). Much maligned, most of the adverse publicity stems from flawed and misinterpreted scientific studies. The family of parabens are naturally occurring chemicals, found mostly in fruits, vegetables and other plants (vanilla pods are especially rich in methyl paraben). Contrary to what is often written, parabens are not especially oestrogenic (not even as much as foods such as carrots or apples, far less than soya). One widely publicised study claimed to find traces of parabens in breast tissue samples, but traces of parabens were also found in their blank control samples (which should have been just that – blank). Speaking to the researcher here, Dr Philippa Darbre, she confirmed that traces of parabens came from the laboratory glassware, probably from the cleaning agents. It is entirely feasible that the parabens 'detected' in the breast cancer tissue samples were also actually present solely due to contamination of the laboratory glassware. No other studies have since found parabens in breast cancer tissue.

Unfortunately, the media's grip on the subject is such that many skincare ranges are now sold as 'parabens-free' as if this were a good thing. In reality, parabens have been tested since the 1930s and have been shown to be safe, highly effective and non-irritating skincare ingredients, so removing them may actually make skincare less safe. Perversely, newer preservatives do not have the same long history of safety testing.

Treating your face

Give yourself a gorgeous facial at home – the full salon treatment without any expense. What's more, it's all performed by the practitioner who knows your skin best – yourself!

Of course it's wonderfully pampering to have a salon facial, but you can also do a great job at home. Just make sure you get everything ready – and ban any interruptions for an hour.

Here's the running order of what to do:
✳ **Cleanse** ✳ **Exfoliate** ✳ **Steam**
✳ **Extractions, if any** ✳ **Tone** ✳ **Mask and rest**
✳ **Facial massage** ✳ **Moisturise**

Cleanse, exfoliate, steam and tone:
After you have cleansed and exfoliated as I have described, start the steaming. It's one of the best ways to prep your skin for a weekly facial treat. (Don't do this, however, if you have very high colour on your cheeks, or rosacea.) You can buy fancy gadgets but I get the best results by steaming my face over a basin of hot water for five minutes.
✳ Fill a bowl with just-boiled water and allow it to cool for a minute or two.
✳ If you haven't already done so, cleanse your face and neck scrupulously, and tie back your hair, or use a soft stretchy hairband.
✳ You can get skin softened and prepped from plain steam, with nothing added to the water, although adding a few drops of essential oil will help blemished or spot-prone skin. All pure essential oils are volatile oil compounds and therefore have antiseptic and antibacterial properties.

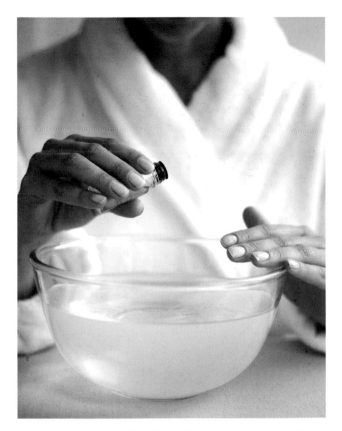

Add a few drops of essential oil to help blemished or spot-prone skin – it's stress-relieving too

My favourites for facial steaming are lavender (good for all skin types), rosemary (for oilier skins) and tea tree (highly antibacterial and thus excellent for helping to purify spots and breakouts). If you have a cold or congested sinuses, use pine and/or eucalyptus essential oil.

✳ Add three to four drops to the water just before you put your face over it, and swoosh round with a toothbrush handle or similar (metal might get too hot). Essential oils are broken down by heat, so drop in at the last moment to retain maximum potency and aroma.

✳ With the towel over your head, take six deep slow breaths (through your mouth may be more comfortable). Move your head a little so every part of your face benefits from the cleansing steam.

✳ Remove the towel after about five minutes and use it to pat the skin dry.

✳ If you need to extract small spots or blackheads, now's the time (see box on right).

✳ Follow with a sweep of skin toner sprinkled onto cotton wool pads to cool the skin.

Extracting small spots or blackheads:

The easiest time to remove any small spots or blackheads is just after steaming when skin is softer. Apply a small dab of plant oil (eg, grapeseed or almond) or balm to the affected area. Wrap both index fingers in a tissue (pull it in half, so you have two thin sheets) and gently press the blemish to unclog the plugs of sebum. Wipe clean and follow with a sweep of skin tonic. If the spot is deep, don't push or poke too hard; it may not be ready to be extracted. A tip: good light is essential and if you don't have 20/20 vision, a magnifying mirror is very useful.

Face mask – and rest...

✳ Apply a generous layer of your favourite mask to both face and neck, but avoid the immediate eye area. Clay-based masks are useful for spot-prone congested skin, whereas creamy, oil-based masks are more nourishing for drier skins. It's fine to mix and match masks and use a richer, hydrating formula on drier cheeks. Apply with your fingertips, or – a little secret – use a blusher brush to paint the mask over your face.

✳ To help you rest and make your eyes sparkle, dampen two cotton wool pads with a little toner or diluted witch hazel (one part with four parts of pure water). If possible, chill the pads in an ice tray for 10 minutes before applying.

✳ Lie down with your feet up – raising your ankles above the level of your heart helps the circulation – and relax for 15–20 minutes.

✳ Remove the eye pads and thoroughly wipe away the mask with a damp muslin cloth, flannel or facial sponge.

Face, neck and shoulder massage with acupressure

This wonderful routine, which takes about ten minutes, comes from renowned international facialist Arezoo Kaviani, who worked with me to devise our Liz Earle Signature Salon Facial. It helps to refresh and rejuvenate your face, at the same time relaxing your mind – which, of course, helps release tension in the facial muscles. It's a perfect part of a home facial, although you can do it separately, too. Try it – it's amazing and really works.

After cleansing, toning and moisturising, sit in front of a mirror in a quiet room with low lighting.

✳ Slow your breathing.

✳ Cup your hands up over your eyes, to rest them and create a sense of darkness.

✳ Eyes closed, bring your hands to your ears and cover them for a few moments until any sounds ebb away, still consciously taking slow deep breaths.

✳ Put one palm over your forehead and the other on the back of your head just above your neck (at the bottom of your skull). Hold firmly for 1–2 minutes (see pic 1).

✳ Keeping the hand on your forehead, move the other and place it over your heart, hold for a few moments, while you think of something that makes you really happy.

✳ Rest your hands lightly on your thighs.

✳ Open your eyes and rotate your neck slowly to loosen your neck muscles: turn your head and look left, then let your neck dip and roll it to the right, and then back to the left. Repeat three times (more if tense), then bring your head to the centre, and rest.

✳ Warm a little plant oil or your favourite facial massage oil (such as apricot kernel oil) in your palms and, with cupped hands, pinch, knead and massage your neck. Work from the bottom of your neck where it meets your shoulders all round the sides and up to the base of the scalp, slowly unknotting any tensions or stress. If you find any sore spots, rotate your fingers over them to relax tight muscles and help ease any pain.

✳ Rotate your shoulders forwards and then backwards for three cycles each, then shake out your arms. Feel your body become softer, the muscles calmed and comfortable.

✳ Warm a little more oil on your palms and sweep your palms, one after the other, up the front of your neck in smooth regular movements.

✳ Using your thumb and forefinger, pinch along your jawbone with firm movements (see pic 2). Then place your middle fingers on the apples of your cheeks and massage this area with circular movements to relieve any tension spots (see pic 3). Open your mouth slightly and let your lower jaw move loosely from side to side.

✳ Press the pads of your thumbs against the sides of your nose at the top and smooth outwards, working your way down the nose. Then, in stages, massage along your cheekbones with your fingertips, using firm circular motions, towards the ears (see pic 4). Be careful not to stretch or pull your skin.

✳ Press against the sides of your nostrils with your middle fingers, sweeping on to your cheeks.

✳ Sweep your palms up the sides of your face, to lift the skin and stimulate circulation.

✳ Starting in the middle, press your thumbs down gently above your eyebrow bones, hold for a moment, then release. Work your way gently along the eyebrow and follow the orbital bone under the eye; repeat four to five times – this helps ease any puffiness.

✳ With eyes closed, gently tap your fingers across your eye sockets, avoiding the tear duct.

✳ Place your thumbs, facing downwards, in the centre of your forehead, between your eyebrows. Sweep your thumbs up and over your eyebrows in an arch-like movement towards your temples, then hold for a moment. Release, then repeat several times (see pic 5).

✳ With your eyes closed, take a deep breath and massage the rims of your ears with your thumbs and the tips of your first two fingers, pressing around the ear lobes up to the top of the ear (see pic 6). Feel the fizz of energy!
FINALLY, refresh the face with a sweep of skin tonic on a cotton wool pad, then lightly massage your favourite moisturiser onto face and neck.

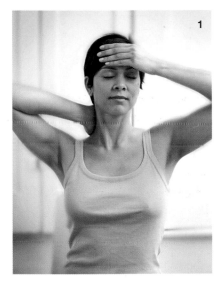

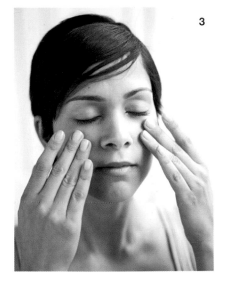

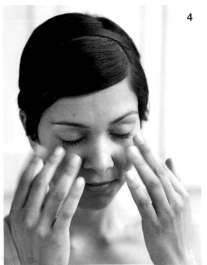

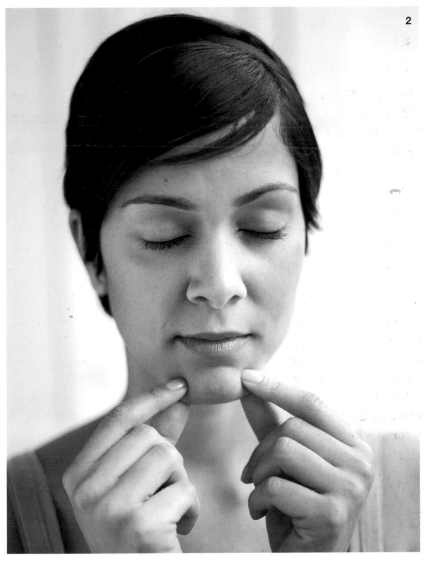

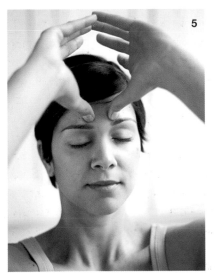

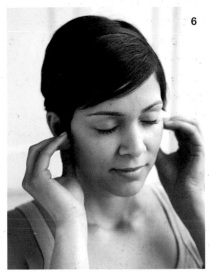

Beautifiers for your body

The best news? It's not rocket science! A little time and attention and, whatever your size and shape, the skin all over your body can be soft, sleek and peachy smooth.

Let's start with body brushing, one of the least expensive (you just need a brush and they last for years) and most rewarding treats you can give your body. As well as removing little lumps and bumps, it encourages lymph to flow freely, helping to perk up your body in general and, in conjunction with a good diet and exercise, to remove pockets of cellulite. It may sound as if it hurts, and those of a sensitive disposition may feel that applying a stiffish bristle brush to dry skin is downright cruel, but you will grow to love it – and the results, of course. All the women I know who have done it for a while absolutely rave about it.

When you choose a brush, look for something you can use easily in either hand. It needs to be stiff enough to create friction, but not to scratch your skin. Ones I like include the Liz Earle version – of course – a natural bristle body brush which has a long (removable) handle, and the Raffe Body Brush by Origins.

Before stepping into the shower, brush the soles of your feet to stimulate blood flow, then work up the lower legs and all over your thighs and buttocks in long, smooth, upward strokes. Continue up your stomach, but don't touch your breasts (the bristles are too harsh). Work up your arms from the wrists to your neck: if you have achy shoulders and/or neck, brushing can really help.

Wherever you are brushing, you want to work towards your heart as this helps the flow of lymph towards the nodes at the heart. Focus on any especially pimply or flabby areas, such as the back of upper arms and buttocks. Don't brush any sensitive areas, or broken skin.

Follow with your favourite body scrub (or make your own, as I sometimes do), working all over your body in the same upwards direction. Then turn on the shower and rinse off. For the brave among you: blast a jet of cold water up and down your body – it's brilliant for helping to tone the backside and breasts by stimulating blood circulation and the flow of lymph.

My favourite salt and oil body scrub

Mix 50ml grapeseed oil with 50g fine sea salt. For a lovely scent that will linger on your skin, add two or three drops of pure essential oil, such as lavender, rose or neroli (orange blossom). Step into a (dry) shower or bathtub and massage the mixture into dry skin, concentrating on any rough patches around knees, elbows, upper arms and heels. Rinse off with warm water before showering or bathing as usual.

Leave your skin slightly damp as this helps to hydrate the skin and apply a generous layer of nourishing body cream (I like products that contain shea butter). Again, always work towards your heart. You may not have the time to exfoliate daily (though I do suggest daily body brushing, if you can), but try to be generous with the body cream – it makes such a difference.

Body hair removal

My favourite method of removing hair from leg and underarms is epilation, which includes waxing, sugaring, threading and lasers, as well as gadgets called epilators. Unlike depilation – where the hair is removed above the skin surface, as in shaving – epilation involves removing the entire hair, including the part below the skin. So epilation keeps skin smoother and stubble-free for longer.

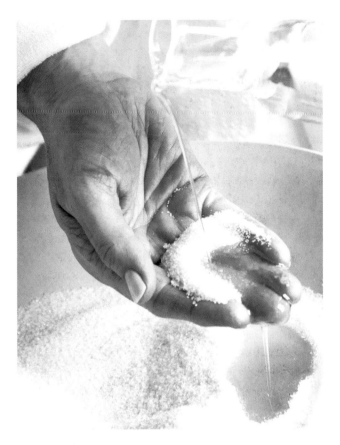

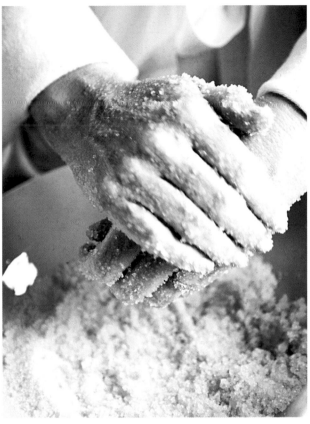

The Iranians invented the process of threading, where hairs are simply tugged out by a piece of cotton thread 'scissored' across the skin; experienced operators are simply phenomenal to watch as they work at tremendous speed, their fingers flashing. Threading is especially good for sensitive areas such as eyebrows, upper lip and bikini line. I also like sugaring or hot waxing for these areas, and underarms and legs: the substance – sugar or wax – is warmed and applied to the skin; then a strip of cotton fabric is pressed on in the direction of the hair growth and whisked in the opposite direction, pulling the hair with it. It's best not to wax around the time of your period, as the skin is super-sensitive and the process is more painful.

I am also a fan of epilating machines, which look a bit like an electric razor. An epilator has blunt rotating teeth that grab the hairs and pluck them out. It's great for underarms and legs, and brave souls could try it on the bikini line and upper lip – you can find mini-epilators which are shaped specially to make these contours easier to cover. Although epilation can be painful the first time you do it, because you

Treat

For serious de-fuzzing, visit a professional salon first, then maintain more sparse re-growth at home. Be sure to exfoliate between hair-removal sessions to help prevent dry skin build-up and ingrowing hairs. Avoid heat treatments of any kind (sunbathing/sauna/steam) for 12 hours before and after waxing, to avoid skin irritation.

have most hair to remove, the re-growth will be consistently more sparse each time, and thus hurts less. Women who have been epilating or waxing for decades say that eventually hair can disappear entirely in some areas. The best version I've tried is the Panasonic ES2067, which can be used wet or dry (wet is less painful).

Back beauty

A satin, smooth-skinned back looks great in a low-cut frock, on the beach or just au naturel.

Body brush: work daily from your thighs to your derrière and on upwards to shoulders to stimulate circulation and banish blemishes. You will need a long-handled brush for this, as mentioned on the page 92.

For spot-prone backs: buy a natural-fibre back strap and use it daily in the shower to gently buff the skin, boosting blood flow and exfoliating simultaneously. Apply a gentle body wash or gel to create a cleansing lather, rinsing well under running water. Use a cotton bud to dab small amounts of antibacterial essential oil onto the affected area (try lavender, melissa or tea tree) and ask a loved one, mother or friend to help with hard-to-reach places.

Apply a mask: recruit a helper to apply a toning or deep-cleansing mask over your back and lie down flat on your tummy for ten minutes to let it work.

Have a back facial: if your budget permits, have a professional back treatment – once a month is ideal, but anything is better than nothing. It can cleanse, remove any little blockages and nourish your back, just as with your face. This is especially good before a holiday in the sun.

Steam it: go for a sauna and/or steam at your local gym, health centre or baths – weekly, if possible – to clear pores and reduce congestion. It's also wonderfully relaxing. Dot spots with a deep-cleansing clay mask before going in to the sauna, to help draw out impurities.

Moisturise: body sprays are the easy way to moisturise the back; use formulations made with pure plant oils on dry skin after bathing. Avoid 'dry oil' sprays, though, as they contain mineral oil and synthetic aerosol propellants that can dry the skin, as well as damage the environment.

Go golden: for those who are pale, a less-than-perfect back will look better if it's lightly tanned. Have a girls-night-in party and get (fake) tanning. (Don't do what a friend of mine did once and apply bronzing powder… it all came off on her beau's white shirt sleeve.)

The bottom line is to move more! We should literally get off our backside to keep it from spreading. It doesn't take much activity: simple things like walking whenever you can or running up and down the stairs can really help.

Treat

If you are in a sauna or steam room, or even your bathroom, add one or two drops of strongly antiseptic eucalyptus oil to the hot coals – or water – to help clear your sinuses and protect against germs.

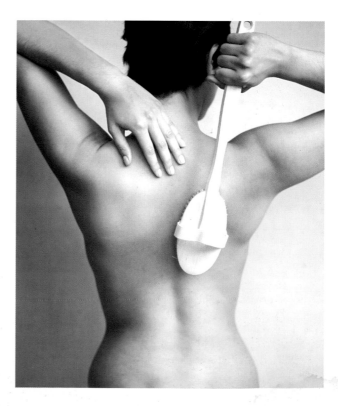

Blissful baths

A long candlelit soak in a scented bath is one of the simplest – yet surest – ways to restore mind and body to restful balance

Using aromatherapy oils turns a simple routine into a treat that benefits both your psyche and your skin. The sense of smell has a powerful influence on your mood and emotions because nerve endings from the brain connect directly with the olfactory channels in the nose. What we smell is transported directly to the limbic system, the part of the brain that is responsible for regulating our emotions. (In fact, the emotional response to an aroma comes before we recognise what it is, which happens in another part of the brain, the cortex.) It's not just feelings that are affected by smell: researchers at Newcastle University in England discovered that rosemary essential oil stimulates the part of the brain that controls hand-eye coordination – so have some on hand to inhale when you need a lift. Lavender, on the other hand, has a physically sedating effect, so is best used at the end of the day to calm and unwind.

To prepare your aromatherapy bath, swirl in a teaspoonful of pure plant oil to soften and smooth the skin – grapeseed, apricot and almond are all good options. Mix your chosen essential oils with a few drops of plant oil (or a little milk or cream – very Cleopatra) and add them once the bath is run: essential oils are broken down by heat and the effect will last longer if you add them just before stepping in.

Tip

Make sure the bath water is not too hot, or it will drain you physically, or even scald the skin. Have a couple of soft fluffy towels warmed on the radiator for when you emerge.

The best body boosting bath

Sitz baths may sound like water torture, but they are a tried and tested health and beauty favourite. Simply run a bath with cold water (yes, just the cold tap!) to about 5cm deep. Sit in the bath with your legs up and over the side. The water should cover your backside and hips, just coming up to your navel. I put on a soft cardigan to keep my top half warm. Stay in the water for 2–3 minutes, then get out and pat skin dry. This is also a good tonic if you have been under stress of any kind. The theory is that the cold water 'shocks' the liver into renewed activity, cleansing the body from within.

These are some of my own favourite combinations of essential oils:

To wake up: 3 drops rosemary and 3 drops neroli, orange or grapefruit

To calm and balance: 3 drops lavender and 3 drops neroli or vetiver

To luxuriate: 3 drops patchouli and 3 drops neroli or rose

To switch off: 3 drops chamomile, 3 drops lavender

I also like to massage oils into the skin when it's still warm after a soak, as the oils are absorbed into the upper layers of the epidermis more rapidly. I am particularly fond of this simple recipe for body oil: combine 100ml grapeseed oil with 5ml (1 teaspoon) wheatgerm oil and 5 drops pure lavender or chamomile essential oil.

Slack attack

Cellulite is fat – medically called subcutaneous fat, located just under the dermis. But cottage-cheese thighs aren't seen only on 'plumptious' beauties: real skinnies can be affected too – even Olympic athletes. Research shows it affects 85 per cent of girls after puberty and over 95 per cent of women over 30, so you're almost odd if you don't have it.

It may not be sizeist, but cellulite is undoubtedly sexist. Men really don't get cellulite. Lobes of fat in the hypodermis (or subcutaneous fat layer) are packed into 'chambers', with walls made of strands of connective tissue (the stretchy collagen and elastin which are responsible for skin tone and tautness). In men, the chambers consist of small diagonal units, whereas in women, they're much bigger, with plenty of room to store an abundance of fat. Cellulite occurs when the blood vessels break down and allow water to leak into the tissue. The fluid accumulates, causing the collagen and elastin fibres to lose their elasticity. At the same time, the clumps of fat begin to migrate upwards, so they can be seen through the skin. As the fibres become taut, they pull down on their anchor points in the top layer of skin, creating the mattress-like puckering and dimpling.

Cellulite is linked to female hormones, predominantly oestrogen: women have bigger fat storage chambers below the waist, which is why cellulite tends to appear on bottoms and thighs. It first manifests in girls going through puberty and seems to be made much worse by taking the contraceptive pill. Oestrogen encourages fluid retention, a key factor in cellulite. Toxins may also be a factor: some organic beauties swear that a pesticide-free diet, among other clean-living measures, keeps their thighs looking smooth.

Experts assess cellulite in four stages. The first, you're fine: your thighs, tum and bum look smooth and when you do the pinch test, there's not a dimple to be seen. At stage two, dimples appear when you pinch a fold of skin between thumbs and forefingers. Further down the line at the third stage, just keep lying down: your skin still looks smooth when you're prone but stand up and the lumps and blobs show all too clearly. By stage four, it doesn't matter what position you're in – the evidence is there.

So what's the solution? To be honest, we're talking improvement here rather than cure. These are the time-tested solutions I recommend:

Stretching and toning exercises undoubtedly help – have you ever seen a dancer or yoga teacher with cellulite?

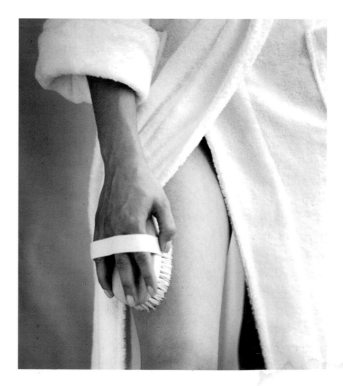

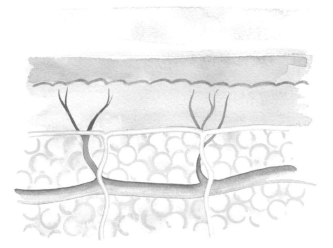

Regular, ordered fat cells in the subcutaneous fat layer keep the skin's surface smooth and dimple-free

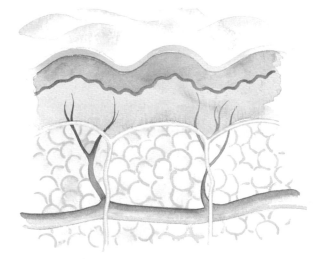

Expanded fat cells, accumulated toxins and fluid retention all contribute to cellulite skin dimpling

Get really in tune with your body and you will be able to 'pull up' your thighs to make them tauter and tighter. (Do the sequences I recommend in chapter 8 regularly – and you should see the difference.)

I'm a big fan of **dry skin body brushing**, which is very effective at dispersing orange peel skin on the surface and sometimes seems to flatten out more serious bumps; more expensively, manual lymphatic drainage massage (from a professional) also encourages sleeker limbs.

Aim to **limit the villains in your diet** – processed foods, white sugar and flour, saturated fats, caffeine and alcohol – for wholesome fresh food including plenty of vegetables, fish, olive oil, eggs, poultry, game, soya, seeds, nuts and nut butters. If you want to lose weight, cut out grains and other carbohydrates such as rice, pasta and potatoes – these carbs become sugar. You can get all the carbs you need from eating vegetables. And eat no more than two pieces of fruit daily, as these are also high in sugars.

Drinking water will help flush out toxins and benefit the functioning of your entire body, speeding the metabolism and assisting the lymphatic system. Herb teas and tisanes can also have a detoxifying effect, particularly nettle, fennel and dandelion, which are diuretic. Supplements of vitamin C and E help strengthen weak cell membranes and collagen, and glucosamine provides the building blocks to repair connective tissue. Rutin may also be useful if you know you're not eating enough vegetables and fruit: this

bioflavonoid (often called vitamin P), which is totally safe, comes from natural sources such as onions, citrus fruit and buckwheat, and may help to prevent the migration of wasted water outside the skin cells, which can result in the dimpling effect. (Don't take rutin without vitamin C, and check with your doctor if you are on antibiotics.)

There are several time-tested **botanical ingredients** for topical use that really do have a skin stimulating and de-puffing effect when applied in hip and thigh gels or creams, including ivy, butcher's broom, horse chestnut (which is useful for the venous system generally) and gingko biloba. Caffeine is a useful anti-cellulite ingredient as it stimulates the skin (as opposed to jangling the central nervous system when consumed). Although none of these will work on their own, they are useful additions to a cellulite-reducing regime.

Anti-cellulite massage oil

Blend 50ml grapeseed oil with five drops each of juniper, cypress, lemon or mandarin essential oils. Shake together in a small bottle and massage into dry skin. This isn't a miracle cure, but massaging twice daily with this skin-toning oil blend will stimulate the circulation and encourage the dispersal of trapped waste matter. It's best applied after using a body scrub in the shower or bath.

Bosom pals

Skin tissue around the bust area is fine and fragile, but specific care can help keep busts in better shape.

Bust firming and toning treatments are useful if your bosom has dramatically changed in size from weight loss or gain, pregnancy and breastfeeding. While it's not possible to rejuvenate stretched skin completely, you can certainly improve its look and tone.

Always take your moisturiser down your chest: it's the most foolproof way to achieve a velvety-soft cleavage.

Your bosom is a suntrap – so unfortunately our décolleté ages fast. Always apply a good SPF20–25 sunscreen when skin is exposed to the elements: even on a grey day, UV light can affect your skin. I even apply a sunscreen to my upper chest when I go out for an early morning walk, as I have seen the price many pay for neglecting this area.

A poorly fitting bra is not only unflattering but may cause broken capillaries under the bust by exerting pressure on the tissue. So get your breasts measured and new bras fitted properly. If you want to wear an underwired bra, try to keep it for high days and holidays rather than everyday use: the wires can dig into the delicate skin tissue. A soft elasticated support is more comfortable for everyday wear, and essential for sport, including the gym.

Massage a nourishing oil, or other specific bust formulation, onto and around your bust daily. As well as keeping the skin in the best condition, rubbing it in under your bosom along the bra line will help prevent broken capillaries building up and encourage the lymphatic system to work more efficiently (vital for breast health). Always massage around each breast towards the armpit in an upward move, and around. Look for specific bust-firming ingredients such as *Kigelia africana*, and extracts of quince and mangosteen. Added skin nourishers such as hyaluronic acid (more on page 43) are beneficial, too – another good reason to take your moisturiser or serum down your bosom. Facial serums often contain excellent

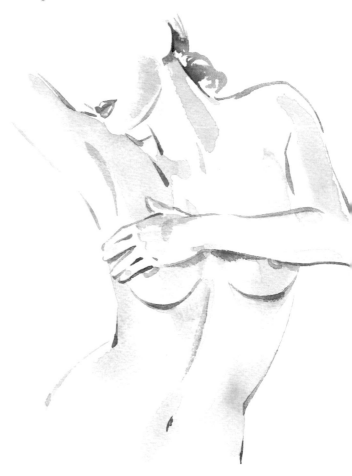

Regular massage also helps detect early formation of breast lumps and cysts

moisturising and skin-firming ingredients and will benefit the bust without the need to buy an extra skincare product.

Directing the shower on your bosom, turned to the coldest you can bear, can really make a difference to the uplift factor! Do it as much as you can. If you like gadgets, try Clarins Model'Bust, a contraption that has been around for years and whizzes cold water around each bosom.

Use a gentle facial exfoliator in the shower (a body scrub is too harsh) to keep skin smooth and pimple free.

Perk up your bustline

Fitness instructor, Viv Worrall, suggests this very simple hand press:

* Sit upright on a chair, or the floor.
* Bring your hands together at chest height: with elbows bent and palms touching, lightly lace fingers.
* Press palms together, as if squeezing a lemon.
* Hold for 2–4 seconds, release, then repeat 8–10 times. This helps strengthen the muscles that keep the breasts from sagging.

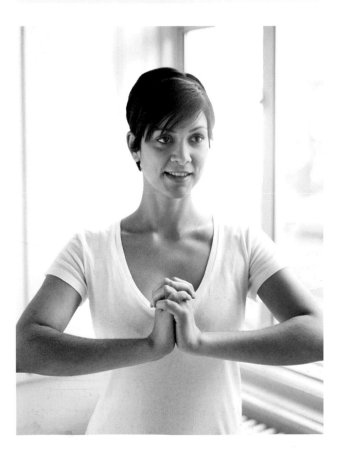

Deodorants – good or bad?

More scares have surrounded underarm toiletries than any others. After researching the topic in detail, both for myself, my daughters and female customers, I find that much of what is written (especially on the web) is needlessly worrying. The family of preservatives known as parabens used in some skincare, though generally not deodorants, does not cause breast cancer by 'migrating' to breast tissue. Studies suggesting this were flawed. My favourite 'deos' are the solid twist-up sticks which dry instantly without causing any stickiness. When I am in mainland Europe I bulk-buy an Italian budget brand called Neutro Roberts: it's inexpensive, works well and has an especially fresh scent. As a simple anti-perspirant, I like the solid 'rock crystal' type that you dip into water and rub against the skin. They leave a film of alum (the mineral salt version of aluminium) and work in much the same way as conventional antiperspirants – temporarily constricting the sweat ducts, so they close up. They are more expensive, but one crystal can last for up to a year, unless you drop it on a hard floor – they shatter!

Regular antiperspirants also contain the mineral salts aluminium chlorohydrate or aluminium zirconium (chemical cousins to the alum-based crystal deos) and some have erroneously linked these with an increased risk of breast cancer. Studies show a small potential for aluminium salts to penetrate into, but not necessarily through, the skin. However, even if a small amount were to be absorbed (eg, through shaving nicks), it would be tiny in comparison to the amounts of aluminium we eat in foods every day. The largest study to date of 1,600 women found no link at all between using deodorants or antiperspirants, either alone or after shaving, with an increased breast cancer risk. The major cancer research charities have all published information discrediting any link between breast cancer and underarm products, including Cancer Research UK, the American Cancer Society and the US National Cancer Institute. A fact sheet called Deodorant, Antiperspirants and Breast Cancer Risk: The Facts is available from Breakthrough Breast Cancer (www.breakthrough.co.uk).

Hands

Keeping hands and feet feeling soft
and looking pretty not only makes us
look smarter but also feels so much
more comfortable.

Unlike our bodies, which are more or less constantly
clothed, our hands are pretty much always exposed to the
elements – notably the sun. Think how hard they work too,
amid an army of aggressors from household cleaners –
particularly the multi-daily dips into detergent – to being
used as paper knives and staple removers.

When I'm a guest on the QVC shopping channel, I
frequently cleanse, tone, exfoliate and moisturise the back
of my left hand as part of a skincare demonstration. I
promise you – by the end of the show, my left hand really
does look ten years younger! I feel like rushing home to do
the other hand.

Giving yourself a manicure at home is one of the simplest
beauty salon treatments – the equivalent of giving yourself
a facial. Ideally, settle down and tend to your hands every
week. If you are really pressed for time, skip the coloured
varnish and just stroke on oil, or sweep on a glaze of clear
varnish. My own favourite is a French manicure, using soft
clear pink varnish tipped with white.

Sugar-scrub recipe

This is my favourite home-spun recipe for softer
skin on hands and feet. Simply mix together two
tablespoons light olive oil (not extra virgin, as this is
too sticky) or grapeseed oil with 2 tablespoons
granulated sugar. Rub this emollient scrub into
hands and feet, focusing on any hardened,
calloused areas. Rinse under warm running water
and pat dry for instantly silky-smooth skin.

You will need:

✳ Nail polish remover: choose a brand without acetone,
which is very harsh and overdries nails (as well as possibly
affecting the people who use it) ✳ Cotton wool pads
✳ Nail scissors or clippers ✳ Emery board or block
✳ Cuticle cream ✳ Rubber hoof stick ✳ Orange sticks
✳ Hand cream ✳ Varnish: base coat, colour, top coat
✳ Nail oil – avocado is excellent

Wash your hands and scrub nails in warm, soapy water,
then dry thoroughly. If you have ingrained dirt, rub with a
lemon half sprinkled with fine table salt. Remove any nail
polish. Trim long nails with nail scissors or clippers; file
smoothly to match the shape of your cuticle (that's the
most flattering). Never 'saw' back and forth, as this
weakens the nail: just file in one direction. After filing, rinse
your fingertips in warm water and pat dry.

Apply a little cuticle cream or oil (or avocado or light olive
oil) around each nail and massage into the cuticle and nail
base. Leave for a few minutes, so the cream or oil can
penetrate then, with the rubber hoof stick, gently push the
cuticle back. If you don't have a stick, wrap a shred of
cotton wool round an orange stick.

Massage a dollop of hand cream into your fingers, palms
and up the wrists and lower arms. Pay particular attention
to the knuckles, rubbing and pulling them to ease any
stiffness. If you have time, spend 5–10 minutes on this; it is
just so relaxing! If you don't have time to sit while you
watch painted nails dry, just wipe off any traces of hand
and cuticle cream, then paint with clear varnish – or
massage a little oil into the nails. If you are going for the full
monty, line up your base coat, nail colour and top coat.
Start with your little finger and apply each one in three
quick strokes, the first down the middle, then one each
side. When the top coat has had a minute to dry, drip a
couple of drops of nail oil (or other plant oil) over the nails
to 'set' the polish. Then wait for at least 10 minutes.

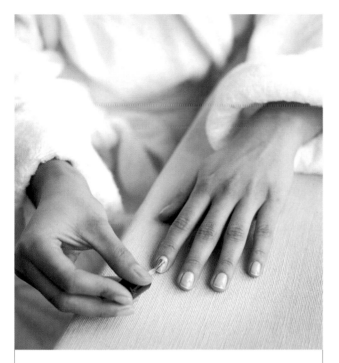

It's vital not to buff weak nails. Buffing removes the top layer of nail and can weaken nails for months in a few seconds. If your nails are split right down, file gently with an emery board, keeping them very short until the splits have grown out; apply oil and hand cream as often as possible.

Wear gloves for every job you can, especially washing up and gardening. Paper absorbs the skin's natural oils, leaving them drier, so working with lots of paper – even reading books – can dry out fingers. Always rehydrate hands and nails with hand cream after washing. If you get a nail nick, file it down immediately, using a glass file if possible – they're the gentlest. I also like the rectangular blocks of nail-buffing foam.

Supplements really can help, but finding the right one isn't always easy. It seems to be a question of what your individual body is missing. Carrying on with the oily theme, there's no doubt that essential fatty acids benefit people who have any deficiency – just as they help hair and skin. Some nails thrive on silica, others on magnesium, zinc or chlorella. Iron deficiency can result in brittle nails: if you suspect this is your problem (you might notice pale lips and eye rims, too), have your iron levels measured; if they are low, consider a gentle supplement such as Spatone or Floradix. If you do take a supplement, take it regularly for at least three months before making a decision about whether it has worked or not. And never use nail varnish remover with acetone if you have weak nails.

On the nail

I've tried many of the more 'natural' water-based brands, but I have yet to find a varnish that isn't dull and doesn't chip or flake off within a day or so. The best results in terms of long-lasting shine come from polishes made with small amounts of toluene and tosylamid or formaldehyde resin. Some may also contain traces of chemicals from the phthalate family; however, despite the warnings you may have read, not all phthalates are the same and those with reprotoxic effects are banned in cosmetic use. But it's true that nail varnish is fairly noxious stuff and you should always apply it in a well ventilated room, preferably near an open window. If you smudge the varnish, lick the tip of your index finger and smooth the polish back into place – but don't actually lick the polish. Or smooth the smudge with a tiny drop of oil. The natural alternative is to buff your nails very gently with a drop of nail oil for brilliant shine. The ranges I have found for good colours, glossy shine and staying power are Jessica, Leighton Denny, Chanel, Essie and Opi.

Secret

Nails love oil, and some of the most expensive 'nail strengthening' treatments are actually little more than a basic plant oil, such as avocado, peach kernel or olive. My tip is to buy a large, inexpensive bottle of one of these and decant into a smaller bottle for your manicure bag. Simply rubbing a dot of oil into the nail bed and surrounding cuticle works wonders to keep nails long, strong and flake-free. Skin balms made with pure plant oils or waxes also work well. Get into the habit of rubbing in a little several times a day, especially during winter months, when hands and nails dehydrate more quickly.

Best feet forward

Love your feet. They work incredibly hard and are miracles of design. If you look after them, they will look after you.

One of my favourite feet treats is a reflexology pedicure, which soothes, comforts and relaxes the whole body. Reflexology is the specific massage or pushing of certain parts of the feet (also the hands and ears) to encourage a beneficial effect on other parts of the body. It sounds strange, but it is one alternative therapy that I believe works. Here are my simple guidelines for a DIY version. (To be on the safe side, don't do the reflexology massage around your lower ankle area if you're pregnant though, as this area is linked to the womb and ovaries.)

Reflexology pedicure:

What you need:

✳ Nail polish remover: choose a brand without nail-drying acetone ✳ Cotton wool pads ✳ Nail scissors or clippers ✳ Emery board or block ✳ Cuticle cream ✳ Rubber hoof stick ✳ Orange sticks ✳ Foot (or hand) cream ✳ Varnish: base coat, colour, topcoat ✳ Nail oil ✳ Toe separators or tissues pleated into bands ✳ Pair of flipflops, fitflops or totally open-toed sandals

Remove any nail polish from toenails.

Start by soaking your feet for at least 5 minutes in a bowl of hot water (or foot spa, if you have one) with two drops of tea tree oil in it, to counter any infections. If you don't have a fancy foot spa/massager, put some marbles in the bottom of the bowl to massage the soles of your feet as you soak.

Wash your feet in the soak, gently scrubbing them with a stiff nail brush and gentle body wash. Then dry them very thoroughly, particularly between the toes, to help prevent fungal infections such as athlete's foot.

Trim long nails by cutting straight across with sharp scissors or toenail clippers. Don't be tempted to cut down

the sides, as nails can regrow into the flesh of the toe and become ingrown. Smooth any rough edges with an emery board or file.

Apply a little cuticle cream or oil and massage it in. With a rubber hoof stick, gently push the cuticles back from the nail bed. Now comes the special part, so make sure you have a good 10 minutes to devote to this:

Start the reflexology on one foot. Massage a nourishing body oil (or olive or wheatgerm oil) into the foot. You can do this in whatever position is most comfortable: the agile can bring the foot they're working on up over the other knee and work on the sole from there. If you are stiffer, you may want to rest your toes on a chair and work from the top.

Use your thumbs and/or knuckles to massage the instep: this covers many points including your adrenal glands, and can really help de-stress you. If you find any sore spots, gently press and hold, releasing after a deep breath in and out.

Treat

Vary your footwear to avoid callouses caused by persistent rubbing. Open-toed sandals are a good option: I like the original Dr Scholl sandal, Birkenstocks, or the more recent, fabulously innovative FitFlops, cleverly designed to exercise foot and leg muscles (thus making foot problems much less likely), sleek your thighs and relieve back ache – they're also extraordinarily comfortable and can be found as sandals, clogs and boots.

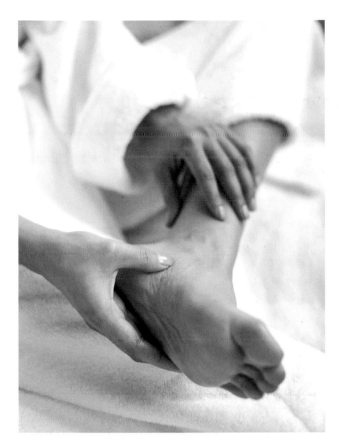

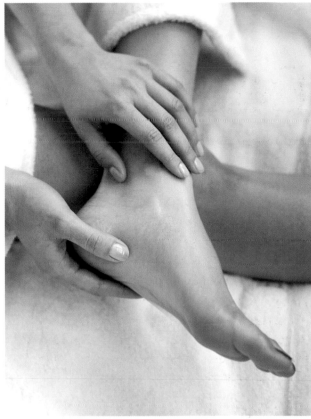

Reflex zones on the feet are linked to specific parts of the body, such as the bladder, spine and pancreas

Gentle, but firm, massage is said to encourage health in these areas

To relieve neck and headaches, press with your thumb on the top of each toe – hold for 5 seconds. When I have a bad headache, I press the tip of my thumb into the back of my big toes, just beneath the fleshy part. Then I move my big toe around, using my thumb and forefinger. Invariably I find a 'crunchy' sore spot, which releases after 30 seconds' gentle massage – and my head clears.

To relieve tension in the sinuses, massage the length of each toe. The reflex zones on this part of the foot are linked to this part of the face. Gently press the underside of each toe upwards.

To boost your whole system: with your thumb, follow the central line down from your second toe to the middle of the ball of your foot. Rest your thumb here, and hold firmly for 5 seconds. This point is linked to the solar plexus, a complex network of nerves central to the body (also a powerful acupuncture point).

To de-stress your back – with your thumb, slowly massage up the inside arch of your foot in little circles. Start at the heel and follow the curve up to your big toe. If you feel any pain or 'crystallisation', rest for 5 seconds on that point.

Once finished, carry on with the rest of the pedicure. If you want to use nail colour, follow the same guidelines as for a manicure, with a base coat, colour (apply in four strokes on the big toes) and topcoat. Remember to stop just short of the cuticles, and the very tips of toenails (so if you bump into anything, the colour won't get damaged). Drip on a little oil after a couple of minutes, pop on the toe separators (or twist tissues in between toes) then sit serenely while they dry.

For a portable massage, you could try a 'footsie roller'. This is a relatively cheap, small, ridged foot massager; you simply remove your shoes and roll your arches back and forth over it, applying extra pressure where required, and it should give instant relief from tension and tiredness.

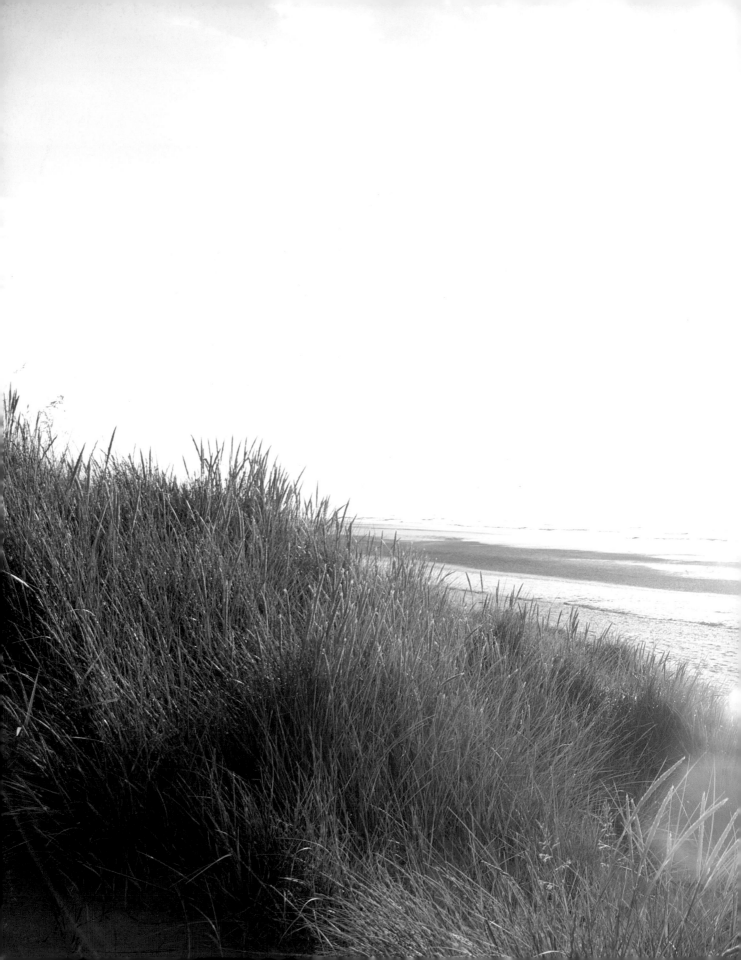

Chapter Five

THE SUN AND YOUR SKIN

I don't obsess about every ultraviolet ray, but I do believe in protecting skin against this powerful force. In this chapter, you'll find simple guidelines for combating the risks – and enjoying the benefits – of the sun.

Golden Moments

A little bit of what you fancy really does do you good.

Contrary to beauty myth, it wasn't Coco Chanel who started the vogue for 'brown is beautiful'. (Apparently she accidentally acquired a tan while on a yacht in the early 1920s and immediately proclaimed it was high fashion.) That may or may not be true, but sunbathing was promoted by doctors in the late Victorian period as a health cure. In one way, they were right. Despite all the downsides of ultraviolet light – sunburn, signs of ageing, inflammatory skin disorders and skin cancers – doctors now agree that brief periods of unprotected sun exposure are among the best natural sources of vitamin D, which helps build healthy bones and reduces the risk of osteoporosis and other diseases, including – paradoxically – skin and other cancers (there's most evidence for bowel, and possibly breast).

Wearing sunscreen blocks the process. But the key is to limit the time. According to the National Osteoporosis Society in the UK, we should bare our face and arms to the sun without sunscreen or clothing only for 15–20 minutes daily or 3–4 times a week, during the summer. Building up your stores in this way gives you enough vitamin D to get through a long, dark winter. More is not better: apart from the other risks, staying in the sun too long without protection means the body breaks down surplus vitamin D shortly after it's produced. Most at risk of low vitamin D levels are those with naturally darker skin (they require more UV exposure to produce enough vitamin D as the pigment in their skin reduces UV absorption), those who wear concealing clothing, office workers or housebound people (especially frail, older ones) and pregnant women. Doctors advise these groups to eat more eggs, meat and oily fish, which supply the best form, vitamin D3 (cholecalciferol) – or take a daily supplement of D3. Anyone who is at particular risk of skin cancer, should do the same. Apart from these vitamin D 'moments', it's vital to protect your skin – and that of your family – so please read on.

Suncare for darker skins

Those with darker skin have more melanin pigment in skin cells and this naturally helps protect the skin from UV damage, resulting in a much lower risk of skin cancer. In fact, if you have this type of skin, you are 10–20 times less likely to develop malignant melanoma, the potentially fatal form of the disease. This doesn't mean never wearing sunscreen: using sun protection has been shown to reduce the risk of non-melanoma skin cancer (basal or squamous cell carcinomas) in African-origin skin. This is important, as the early signs of skin cancers (such as pigment change) in darker skins are more easily missed, making successful treatment harder. Do see your doctor if you notice any change in a mole, freckle or normal patch of skin that occurs quickly – over weeks or months. In particular, check the soles of your feet and the palms of your hands, the most common sites for skin cancer for those with darker skin tones. Using sunscreens will definitely help reduce UV-related skin ageing, and you should reach for these when the local weather UV index is high (level 7, or above).

If you have darker-coloured skin, but have lived for many years in a cooler climate (like the UK), don't assume that your genetic inheritance will protect you if you return to a hot country. Your skin may get burnt, leading to soreness and peeling, because it has become accustomed to a different climate. So it's always better to err on the side of caution.

Because mineral screens (titanium dioxide and zinc oxide) can look ashy on darker skins, choose products based on ultra-fine 'nano' particles, which should provide an effective but invisible screen.

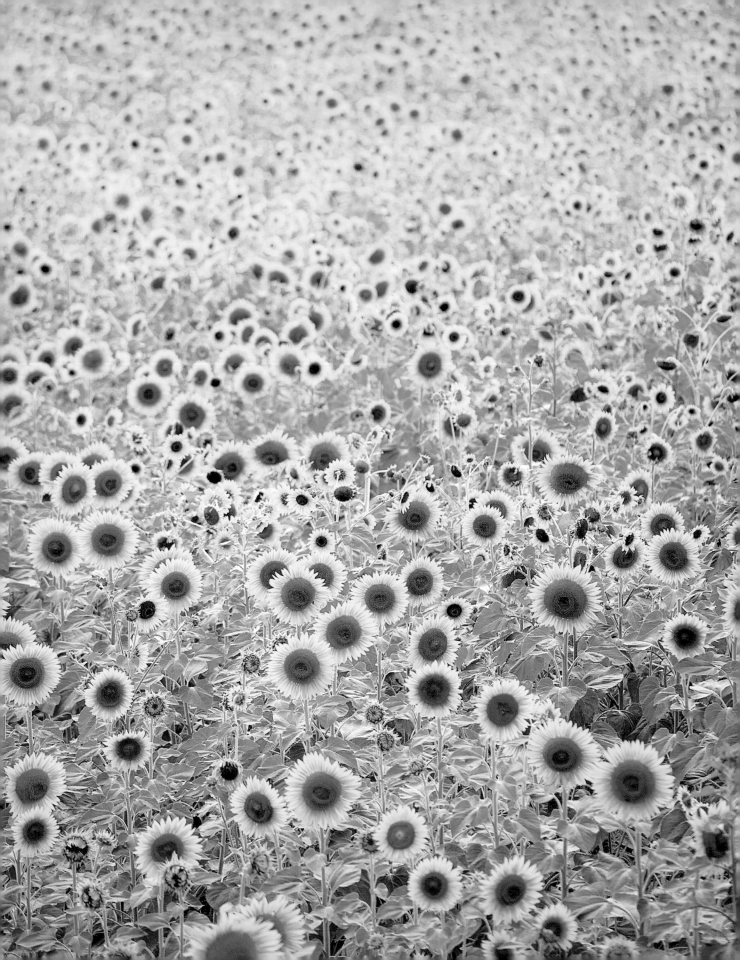

The sun and your skin

Before you make any decisions about exposing your skin to sunlight, it's a good idea to know what it is you are exposing yourself to and how resistant – or not – your own skin (and that of your family) is to this natural force, which offers both health benefits and dangers.

Sunlight is the total spectrum of electromagnetic radiation coming from the sun. It is divided into three wavelengths: UVA, UVB and UVC. All of the UVC is filtered out by the atmosphere, but UVA and UVB radiation both reach the earth in significant amounts. Remember: radiation burns. So exposing your skin to the sun is like grilling a chop or roasting a joint. UVA is the longest wavelength, which penetrates deep into the skin – reaching the dermis – and causes skin 'ageing' and cancer. It even passes through glass, so sitting in your car or by a window in the daylight without sunscreen puts your skin in peril. UVB, which reaches only the epidermis, causes sunBurn (think 'B' for burning) and skin cancer.

A tan is actually a sign that the skin has been damaged and is trying to protect itself by producing melanocytes (pigment cells) to try to absorb further UV radiation. Sun damage causes oxidative stress (see page 14), and degrades the all-important collagen and elastin in the dermis, which makes our skin sag and lose its bounce.

Skin cancer is the fastest growing cancer in the UK, with 75,000 new cases every year, and over 2,300 deaths. The average age of diagnosis is 50 years old, but 20 per cent of cases now occur in young adults, with more among women than men. There are two types of skin cancer, both slow-growing: malignant melanoma, which can be fatal, and non-melanoma skin cancer – which includes basal cell or squamous cell – which is the most common, and can be disfiguring. Basal cell carcinoma usually starts as a small,

Your burn risk

These skin types categorise your `burn risk' – that is, how vulnerable you are to UV rays of the sun. Type I has the lowest amount of protective melanin in the skin and therefore the highest burn risk, and Type VI the lowest burn risk.

Type I – Very fair skin: Tends to have freckles (high density are the most vulnerable), red or very light blond hair, blue or green eyes. Burns very easily, almost never tans. Skin will be badly damaged if exposed to UV light without protection. Redheads and other Type Is have an inefficient type of melanin (pheomelanin) and should always protect themselves completely.

Type II – Fair skin: Tends to have blond or light brown hair, blue or brown eyes. Skin always burns, but also tans slightly. Some people of Celtic origin have Type I or II skin with black hair. Types II to VI have a more efficient and protective type of melanin (eumelanin).

Type III – Light olive skin: Tends to have brown hair and brown or green eyes. Sometimes burns, usually tans.

Type IV – Darker olive skin: Rarely burns, tans easily. Tends to have dark brown eyes and hair. Can still suffer from UV damage; less likely to develop melanoma than Types I to III, but skin will age with sun exposure.

Type V – Brown to light black skin: Often with dark brown eyes and hair. Not as vulnerable to UV-related ageing or skin cancer, but still needs sunscreen during intense or prolonged exposure.

Type VI – Darker black-brown skin: With black-brown eyes and hair. Does not burn easily, but should still use sunscreen to reduce skin ageing.

pale, rounded or flat lump, while squamous cell carcinoma takes the form of red scaly spots or sores. Although slow-growing and easily treated, non-melanoma skin cancers can be fatal, so they must be diagnosed and treated.

People with the highest risk of malignant melanoma (ten times above average) are those with a very large number of normal moles, any number of atypical moles and/or two or more cases of melanoma in first-degree relatives. People with freckles, red or blond hair, skin that burns in the sun and/or any family history of malignant melanoma have two to three times higher risk. These groups must always protect themselves from the sun's rays – so, rather than risking unprotected exposure for the sake of vitamin D production, experts recommend that people in these groups should take a supplement.

Checking your moles

Malignant melanoma usually develops from an existing mole. If it's diagnosed and treated early, melanoma can be cured in the vast majority of cases.

Experts have devised this A, B, C, D, E guide to checking moles:

A is for Asymmetry: both halves of a mole should be the same shape. See your doctor/specialist clinic if a mole starts to change shape and be asymmetric.
B is for Borders: moles should have smooth borders. See your doctor/specialist clinic if you have a mole with irregular or jagged edges.
C is for Colour: a mole should only have one colour. See your doctor/specialist clinic if it has two or more colours – dark brown, light brown and/or pink.
D stands for Diameter: see your doctor/specialist clinic if a mole is more than 6mm in diameter.
E is for Evolution: if a new mole evolves abnormally – ie, grows quickly, or changes in shape and colour, or itches or bleeds – see your doctor/specialist clinic.

Experts also advise consulting a doctor if there is a new, pigmented line in a finger- or toenail (usually thumb or big toe), or something growing under a nail, especially if it's pigmented or bleeding.

Precancerous spots – solar keratoses

Lighter skin types may have developed solar (or actinic) keratoses after repeated minor sun damage over years. They are small, rough, slightly raised bumps, ranging from the size of a pinhead 2–3cm across, usually on the face, neck, backs of hands, bald patch and other areas often exposed to the sun. Their colour varies widely: they can be light, dark, pink, red, the same colour as your skin, or a combination. Some may have a yellow-white crust on top. Sometimes several join together, forming a big rough patch of skin. In themselves they're not dangerous, but around one in ten develops into a squamous cell carcinoma. They're also a warning sign that skin has been under sun assault, so it's important to check for melanoma. The vast majority of solar keratoses – 19 out of 20 – disappear on their own or never progress, but since you can't predict which, they should all be treated, usually by topical drugs, cryotherapy (freezing) or laser.

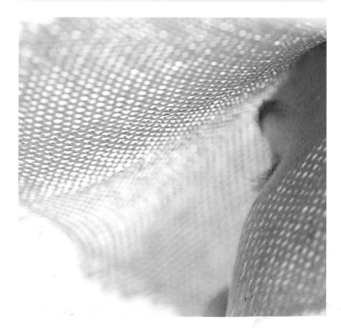

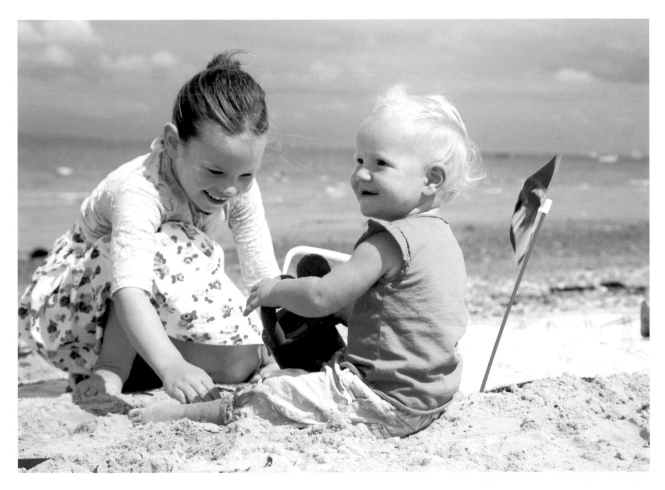

How to protect yourself and your family

While I am not obsessive about avoiding every ultraviolet ray, I agree with dermatologists and UV-radiation experts that we must be sensible when dealing with such a powerful force as the sun. That applies to every one of us – and particularly to fair-skinned children. Little ones spend more time playing outdoors than adults and seeing them running round, getting redder and redder, is so worrying. A severe sunburn when you're young can lead to cancer as a grownup.

Covering up is the first line of defence in strong sunshine. I always have a big hat with a wide brim (every 2.5cm of brim gives you an extra SPF5), closely woven dark clothing (I like cool Kenyan kikoi scarves wrapped round my neck and upper chest, or as a sarong) and lots of sun cream.

There are funky ranges of sun-protective clothing for kids, including caps with peaks and legionnaire back flaps, vital for protecting the vulnerable ears and neck area.

I try to stay in the shade around the midday hours, when the sun is at its highest, as about 50 per cent of the day's UV rays occur then. And I usher my children along with me: games, books and lunch are a good thing to occupy everyone. You can still get tanned – but avoid danger – by sunning yourself at the gentler beginning and end of the day's rays.

Using the right type of sun cream is crucial. I only ever use a sun cream with a physical barrier, such as a blend of the minerals titanium and zinc oxide, which give broad-spectrum UVA/UVB coverage. These minerals stay on the surface of the skin and act as a superfine protective veil, literally bouncing the rays away from the skin.

The minerals can now be micronised (ground up) so finely that they don't leave a chalky coating. Some of these physical sunscreens use cosmetic nano-technology, which makes the particles so small they're invisible, but not so tiny that they penetrate through the upper (stratum corneum) layer of the skin. The particle size of titanium dioxide falls between 20 and 100nm and despite scary headlines, extensive testing doesn't seem to show nano-particles penetrating into the bloodstream. The skin successfully keeps tiny water molecules out – and nano-particles are huge by comparison. More than 16 significant studies around the world between 1996–2008 all show no permeation of nano-particles. An interesting review can be downloaded from http://www.colipa.eu/nanotechnology.html. However, synthetic chemical sunscreens such as the cinnamate and benzophenone families may be an issue as they can irritate and I speak to many who find these chemicals trigger prickly heat and other sensitised skin disorders. (Watch out for the many variations on 'cinnamate' and 'benzophenone' on the ingredient list and avoid them, where possible.)

But synthetic chemical sunscreens may do more than trigger sensitivity. According to research in 2007 from the University of California, they may also generate compounds that attack skin cells. This could not only be dangerous in terms of skin cancer (which, of course, they are intended to prevent), but is likely to increase the visible signs of ageing. The danger occurs, say researchers, when the chemical filters penetrate into the deeper layers of the epidermis, where they can generate harmful compounds called ROS or reactive oxygen species (oxygen free radicals) if they are exposed to ultraviolet light. However, they are less likely to do this if there is still plenty of sunscreen on the skin filtering out the ultraviolet rays. So, if you do use a synthetic chemical sunscreen, you must go on applying it generously every two hours and always when you come out of water or have towelled down. Given the risks of skin sensitivity with multiple applications, I strongly suggest using only a mineral-based sunscreen, especially if your skin is very fair or sensitive, or if you're using it on children.

Faking it

There are more and better self-tanners on the market these days. The principal ingredient in all formulations is dihydroxyacetone which, although a synthetic molecule, may be derived from natural sources. Exfoliate the skin before using any self-tanner to remove the dead skin cells that can make the end result look patchy. Also apply plenty of moisturiser to make sure your self-tanning product glides smoothly on to the skin. I prefer spray versions that

Slap on the sunscreen

Research shows that most of us apply only about half as much sunscreen as we should, and too late. This is one case where more is better: 6 teaspoonsful is about right for a normal adult body. Currently when you choose a sunscreen, remember that the SPF number assesses UVB protection, while UVA protection is generally indicated by the number of stars * the product has, with 1* being low protection and 5* being high. There are new guidelines from the EU which we expect to become legislation in the near future and you can expect to see some changes in the way sun products are labelled. The general levels of protection have been divided into 4 bands: low, medium, high and very high. The low band includes SPF6 and SPF 10, medium band SPF15, SPF20 and SPF25, high band SPF30 and SPF50, and very high band is just SPF50+. In each case, the claimed SPF is the minimum performance except for the SPF50+ category where the minimum performance should be SPF60. In each case the level of UVA screening should be a minimum of one third of the (claimed) UVB screening.

Apply a sunscreen 20–30 minutes before you go out in the sun. Then re-apply 20–30 minutes later. Two thinner (but not skimpy) coats cover better than one thick layer. Add extra onto faces, ear tips, back of necks and legs, which burn easily. Re-apply after swimming, perspiring and towelling dry.

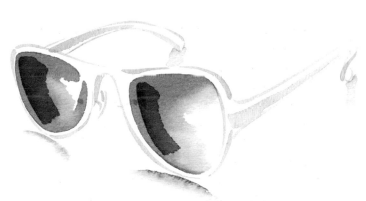

lightly mist the skin and are easier to use on your back and other hard-to-reach places. I also like 60 Second Instant Miracle Tan by Diana B, which I discovered on a trip to sun-worshipping Miami: you simply rub the chocolatey foam all over damp skin and shower off a minute later.

To give your face a natural-looking glow, put a little moisturiser in your hand, add a squirt of self-tan, mix together, and smooth over face and neck. And don't forget to wash your palms thoroughly afterwards.

Sunbeds (although I confess to having used these) are not a safe alternative, according to Cancer Research UK. Excessive use is estimated to cause around 100 deaths from malignant melanoma every year in the UK.

Sunglasses

Too much exposure to intense sunlight can burn the surface of the eye and may seriously damage our sight. Experts say that cataracts, age-related blindness (macular degeneration) and cancer of the eyelids and skin around the eyes are linked to UV exposure. As the ozone layer, which should filter out UV rays, declines, so the effect is intensified. You don't have to be basking on a sunny beach: even light reflected off the pavement may be dangerous, and UV light is strongest when it's reflected off snow, sand and water. So my message is simple: wear sunglasses that are 100 per cent UV protective, the bigger the better. Light can filter round the sides of glasses, so make sure they fit closely to your face and have big arms. Inexpensive sunglasses are fine, as long as they meet these criteria. Polarised lenses reduce glare, so are useful for sailing, and give a better clarity of vision, so are also good for driving.

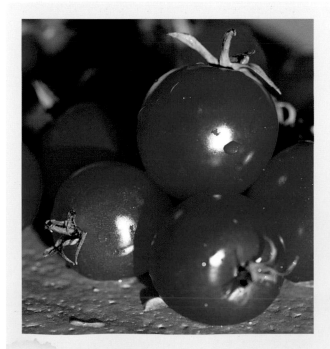

Now eat your tomatoes!

A 'tomato diet' could help prevent sunburn and UV-linked skin ageing, according to a small study by researchers at the Universities of Newcastle and Manchester. People given 5 tablespoons of tomato paste with 10g olive oil daily showed significant improvements in their skin's ability to protect itself against UV rays. Not only did it reduce sunburn, compared to the control group – who were given just olive oil – the tomato diet boosted the level of 'procollagen', a molecule which gives skin elasticity and structure. The key compound is lycopene, the bright red pigment in tomatoes, a powerful antioxidant which neutralises the free radicals that cause much of the sun's skin damage. Tomatoes won't replace sun creams, but may be a valuable addition to the ranks of skin savers.

Keep on glowing

Here are my hints on how to achieve the safest golden glow to last long after sundown.

A little bit of thoughtful preparation goes a long way when you're off on a sunny holiday. A week or two before you go, have your hair cut (and coloured, if you like). And, while we're on the subject of hair, do remember that it will dry out in the sun, just like your skin – more so, if you have colour. So take lots of nourishing hair conditioners and masks – and lavish on oils if you like them. Buy a big-brimmed, closely woven hat to protect not only your face from the sun's rays, but your hair, too (especially if you tuck it up inside). Then get rid of unwanted hair, with a general de-fuzz, including along your bikini line: a useful tip is to breathe in as the therapist applies the wax, then exhale as she strips it off – the ouch factor is greatly reduced.

If your budget permits, invest in a good pedicure to show off bare feet in strappy sandals, or give yourself one (see my suggestions on page 102). A French manicure, with translucent, palest pink varnish and white tips, looks pretty with open-toed sandals, or choose zingy pink or coral to set off your skintone.

And start the fake tanning process (see pages 112-3) a few days before you go, so you can assess the clothes to pack! Don't forget your all-over sun screen, plus a higher SPF for face, neck and décolleté.

For daytime, you need the barest minimum of make-up, but for evenings you might want to glam up a bit…

Daytime

I actually use foundation and bronzing powder when I'm in the sun, partly to give an instant tanned look, but also to top up UV protection by providing additional layers of physical sunblock. (I've successfully used this technique when I was filming in the hottest Caribbean sun.) If you prefer a lighter finish on the skin, a tinted moisturiser will give a little colour and even skintone.

Lips: do wear something on your lips and keep it topped up to protect them against the sun. I wear Liz Earle Sheer Pink Lip Shimmer, which gives a slick of colour – and also comes in gold. I also like lip glosses in bright corals and pinks – young, happy colours! My favourite brands are Stila and Chanel. Even lipgloss provides a little SPF if it has a coloured pigment.

Evening

Perversely, I tend not to wear foundation in the evenings, as skin doesn't need the sun protection. But I do use a skin shimmer such as Nuxe Huile Prodigieuse Golden Shimmer Dry Oil on my temples, cheeks, brown bones, collarbones, legs, décolleté – everywhere, really! MAC also make a lovely formula called Mineralise Skin Finish. And, of course, I use Liz Earle Gold Shimmer.

Sheer bronze highlighter: I use Nars stick bronzer – called The Multiple – on eyelids and brow bones, cheeks, lips, and to highlight cleavage and shoulders (Orgasm is an especially fabulous all-round shade).

Waterproof mascara: my favourite Lancôme Definicils comes in a waterproof version, but I tend just to do my top lashes to prevent 'panda' smudging.

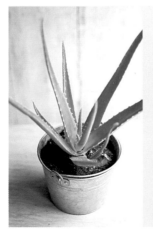

Aloe vera

Aloe vera is a wonderful natural after-sun. If you happen to have the real plant, just snap off a leaf and rub the sap over your skin. Or, choose an after-sun product based on aloe. (Check *Aloe barbadensis* is the first ingredient.)

Skincare in the sun

With the extra layers of sun cream and (if you're like me) make-up, it's as important as ever to use a good cream-based cleanser. Remove it with a muslin cloth or flannel wrung out in warm water: simply the most efficient way to remove gunk and grime. You may like to keep your skin tonic in the fridge for a refreshing reviver in the heat. I also switch to a lighter, more matt, moisturiser to avoid shiny skin in the sun.

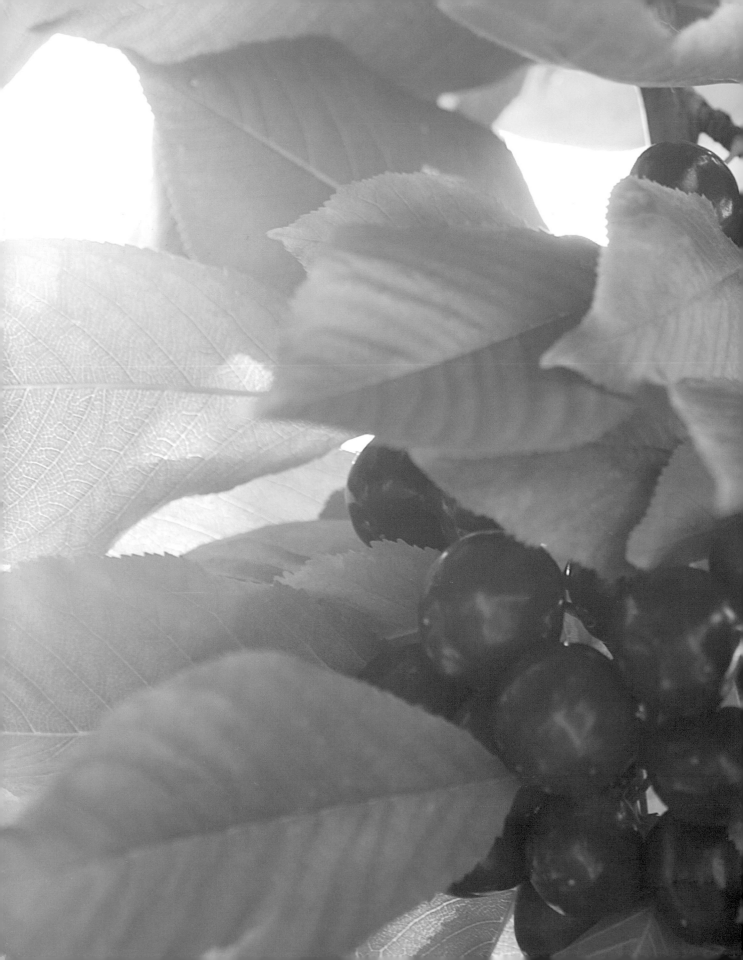

Chapter Six

SKIN PROBLEMS AND SOLUTIONS

Blemished skin is distressing – as I know,
from my own experience of eczema – but there
are many helpful natural remedies for skin
conditions of all kinds, which I detail in
this chapter

Understanding inflammation

Some of the most distressing skin conditions – eczema, psoriasis, acne and rosacea, as well as sensitivity – have in common one underlying factor: out-of-control inflammation.

If you bruise your knee, get sunburnt or catch a cold, the body's immune system deals with it by creating its own 'fire', with heat, redness, pain and swelling. This stimulates the body to marshal its forces, repel the invader and repair the damage. The mechanism has allowed human beings to survive by counteracting disease-causing bacteria, viruses, parasites and toxins. So far, so good: we obviously need the inflammatory response. But many medical researchers now believe that the inflammatory response is running riot and wreaking havoc, mainly due to factors in modern life. Chronic low-grade inflammation is thought by many researchers to be the underlying cause of conditions including heart disease and cancer, asthma, gum disease and even dementia, as well as skin problems.

According to Dr Andrew Weil of the University of Arizona, one of the world's leading experts in integrated medicine, 'What often tips the scales in favour of chronic inflammation are lifestyle factors such as diets high in the wrong kinds of carbohydrates and fats, obesity, inactivity and stress, which can all promote inflammatory reactions in the body. Smoking, high blood pressure, lack of sleep and exposure to toxic chemicals and air pollutants can also increase chronic inflammation. Even getting older seems to stack the deck in favour of inflammation because, over time, the body produces more inflammatory compounds and fewer substances that protect against it. And when long-term inflammation is present, changes can occur on a cellular level that can make you more vulnerable to disease,' he says.

Throughout this book, the advice I am sharing with you will help counter harmful inflammation. In this chapter, you will find specific natural recommendations for different problems, based on research, and advice from clinicians including pharmacist Shabir Daya, who specialises in natural remedies. There are also general guidelines, however, which I outline next, as they are common to all inflammatory skin conditions – and should also be of benefit to the way we look and feel in general.

Don't reject conventional medicine (such as a short course of topical steroids) to get an acute problem under control, before looking to stabilise the skin with a more natural approach. If necessary, ask your doctor for a referral to a dermatologist. Sometimes I use conventional medicine first and then add more natural back-up.

What often tips the scales in favour of chronic inflammation are lifestyle factors such as diets high in the wrong kinds of carbohydrates and fats

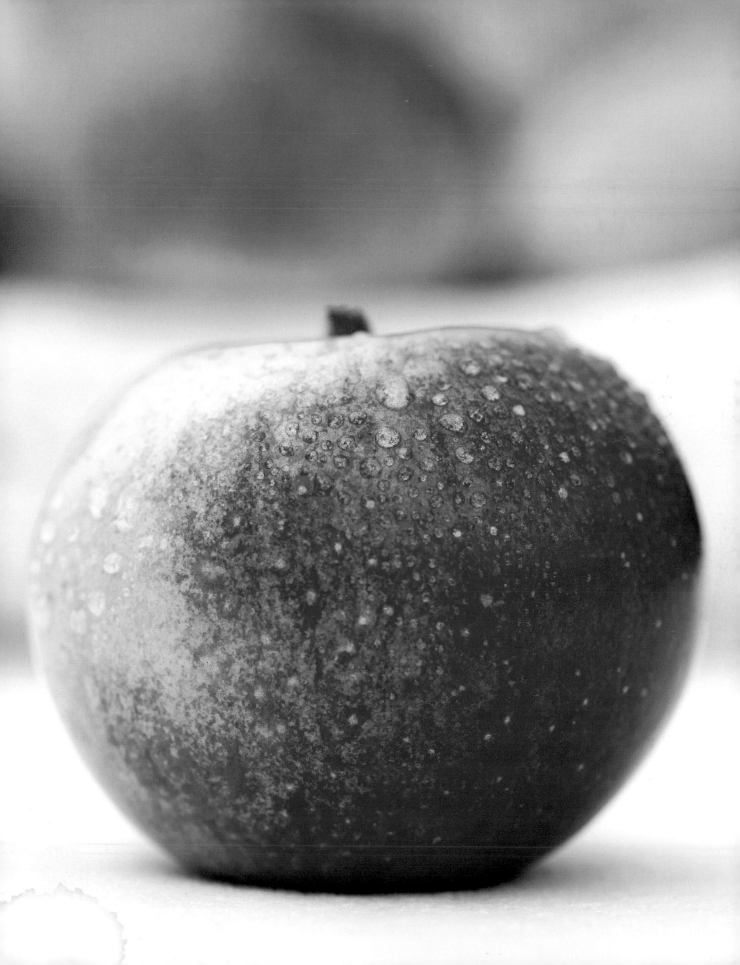

General guidelines for treating problem skin

Eat an anti-inflammatory diet: the low carbohydrate diet I detail in chapter 7, rich in oily fish and an antioxidant-rich range of different-coloured fresh vegetables, salads and fruit, will help reduce inflammation (antioxidants act by preventing oxidative stress, a cause of inflammation). Explore food sensitivities and allergies: the gluten in grains, particularly wheat, and casein in cow's milk can cause inflammation in some people, particularly if their system tends to be inflammatory anyway. It may be worth a trial period eliminating these foods singly, to see if you benefit.

Treat constipation: elimination of toxins from the body is essential to skin health, so avoiding constipation (also a sign of an inflamed gut) is vital. Eat plenty of fibre-rich vegetables and fruit and keep your liver healthy to maintain bowel regularity by ensuring a steady supply of bile salts. Simple but effective liver detoxifiers include bitter-tasting herbs such as milk thistle (*silybum marianum*), dandelion root (*taraxacum officinale*), globe artichoke leaf extract (*cynara scolymus*), Swedish bitters – or even a tot of vermouth or Campari before a meal.

Take appropriate supplements:

Omega-3 essential fatty acids: restoring the right balance of omega-3 and omega-6 fatty acids is essential to making the body less inflammatory (see page 144). As well as eating oily fish and other foods containing omega-3s, consider a supplement of fish oils or, for vegetarians, a supplement derived from algae.

Probiotics: two thirds of the body's immune receptor cells are found in the gut; normalising the balance of gut bacteria by taking a good probiotic supplement (rather than a probiotic drink, most of which contain sugar) is seen as crucial, because an excess of 'bad' gut bacteria is linked to inflammatory conditions, including the very common Irritable Bowel Syndrome. Inflammatory gut problems are inextricably linked with unhealthy skin.

Zinc: this important anti-inflammatory mineral is often deficient in people with inflammatory skin conditions; the immune system is adversely affected by even moderate degrees of zinc deficiency, according to the American Office of Dietary Supplements. (Take as zinc picolinate, for the best absorption.) Good food sources are animal protein, almonds, grains and seeds.

Skincare

Damaged or sensitive skin needs the gentlest care and my advice is to keep it simple, minimising your exposure to common irritants and sensitisers, such as fragrance (including essential oils), synthetic chemical sunscreens and the petrochemical detergents sodium lauryl and laureth sulphates. Fragrance is not only found in skincare, but can settle on the skin from other sources, too, such as body sprays, hairsprays and aerosol air fresheners, so avoid these as well if your skin is suffering.

I recommend reducing your skincare to two basics: a detergent-free (non-foaming) cleanser – preferably removed with a soft muslin cloth, for gentlest daily exfoliation – and a good fragrance-and-sunscreen-free moisturiser.

Some natural skin calmers can help to soothe and heal (such as aloe vera, chamomile, cucumber and calendula) but even natural ingredients may further upset angry skin, as natural chemicals are no less sensitising than synthetic ones – hence the avoidance of essential oils. Some unusual natural remedies may help – I've heard of organic full-fat milk helping to alleviate rosacea for example, but always patch-test anything new by applying to a small area in a less visible place (such as the back of the neck or inner arm) for at least 24 hours before using on your face.

If you're using a cotton muslin cloth to remove cleanser, make sure it's really clean, but check that no detergent residues are left in the cloth, as these will exacerbate the condition. I like washing aids such as Ecozone Wash Balls, which cut out the need for laundry liquids (better for the environment, and cheaper, too), or you can simply boil clothing in plain water to clean it without detergent. If your skin is irritated or broken, buy products with preservatives as the bacteria that breed in non-preserved creams will make damaged skin worse. Preservatives that may be included are phenoxyethanol, parabens, benzoic acid, dehydroacetic acid and polyaminopropyl biguanide. I don't advocate formaldehyde or formaldehyde-forming (when they mix with other chemicals they make formaldehyde) preservatives such as imidazolidinyl urea, diazolidinyl urea, quaternium 15 and DMDM hydantoin. And try not to put your fingers, and their bacteria, into pots: use fresh cotton buds to scoop out instead.

Chlorella – the great green food

Nutritionist Nadia Brydon gave me this recipe for a delicious green smoothie, incorporating chorella, one of the most ancient living organisms (she suggests using the Japanese brand Sun Chlorella). Chlorella is actually a food, not a supplement, and contains an abundance of chlorophyll (pure plant protein), amino acids, various vitamins and minerals. According to Nadia, 'It repairs damaged skin and promotes healthy new cells. It helps the liver detoxify, and also improves digestion and constipation. Chlorella combats inflammation by reducing the acid in your body, making it an alkaline environment, which is much less friendly to bacteria and other invaders.' As well as helping to alleviate skin problems, chlorella has been credited by women I know with producing big improvements in tone and texture. One beauty editor in her fifties describes the improvement as, 'amazing!'.

Chlorella smoothie

Blend together and sip slowly as one dose (or meal replacement) or drink half, refrigerate the rest and drink no later than the same night.

* **1–2 cups of water**
* **½ cucumber**
* **1–2 celery sticks**
* **1–2 parsley sprigs**
* **3–6g chlorella (start with the lower amount and work up gradually)**
* **1 garlic clove**
* **A few leaves basil**
* **Thumbnail-sized piece of fresh ginger, peeled**
* **½ avocado – tasty and contains omega-3 oils**
Himalayan salt to taste (contains 81 minerals)
Fresh ground black pepper
For a sweet-tasting smoothie: omit garlic, salt and pepper, and add half a peeled mango or papaya and/or 1 or 2 raw beetroot, topped and tailed but not peeled (but cleaned!). You can use other greens if you wish.

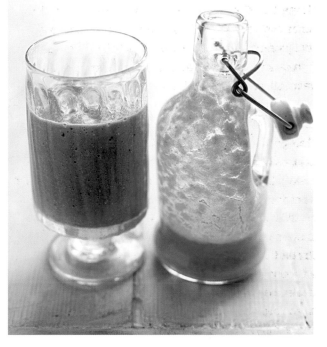

Eczema

This chronic skin disorder is due to a hypersensitivity reaction (that may be an allergy), which leads to long-term inflammation. This manifests in a range of problems, very often itchy rashes, which may be red, scaly, dry and/or leathery. Sometimes the skin becomes blistery, and may become weepy, oozy and/or crusty. There are many different types of this condition, including atopic eczema (sometimes called atopic dermatitis, which runs in families and may be associated with the other atopic conditions, hayfever and asthma) and discoid eczema (disc-shaped lesions, which may weep). Eczema is very common in babies and small children, but many grow out of it.

The problem is not so much the condition as what it leads the sufferer to do – that is, to scratch the itch. It was my own eczema that led me to investigate the emollient qualities of plant oils, which can help stop the itch. Conventional treatment usually involves steroid creams to suppress the inflammation. These may work for a time, but the skin can become tolerant to them, so you need to use more and more, which may damage the skin barrier and make the problem worse. Today, I keep a small tube of steroid ointment in the first aid box and use it sparingly and only when absolutely essential.

I must emphasise that what works for one person may not work for another, but there will be something that helps, so do keep trying. The lifestyle guidelines are also really important for maintaining improvement. Covering every option would take another book, so please do look at the websites of national support programmes (see the Directory).

Red clover is a traditional blood purifying herb prescribed by medicinal herbalists for skin disorders, including eczema

Natural prescription (see pages 186–7)

Try blood-purifying herbs such as red clover, dandelion, burdock and sarsaparilla. These help to eliminate toxins in the bloodstream which appear to trigger inflammation.

Essential Fatty Acids (EFAs) play a vital role in restoring the lipid levels within the outer cells, helping to prevent flaking and dry skin. They also have natural anti-inflammatory properties. Flax seed oil, hemp seed oil, evening primrose seed oil and borage seed oil are all good sources, and can be found combined together in some formulations.

Topical creams can soothe inflamed skin and help prevent itching. Look for products containing plant oils (flax seed, hemp seed, evening primrose oil and borage), with extracts of herbs such as echinacea, red clover, chamomile and nettle. Calendula is a trusted botanical which has improved many skin problems. Relief is found from products based on manuka honey, a staple of traditional medicine in New Zealand and now respected worldwide for its antibacterial, anti-inflammatory and skin repairing properties. The oat grain contains lipids and compounds called avenanthramides, which have a wide range of actions against inflamed, itchy skin; there is some research and much anecdotal evidence for the efficacy of oat-based products. Topical gels containing 2 per cent anti-inflammatory liquorice have been shown to reduce redness, swelling and itching. (Liquorice-based products are also used to heal cold sores.)

This is one of the few times I would suggest using plain Vaseline or petroleum jelly, as it is inert and won't upset even the most sensitive skin (which might react to one of the natural chemicals in plant

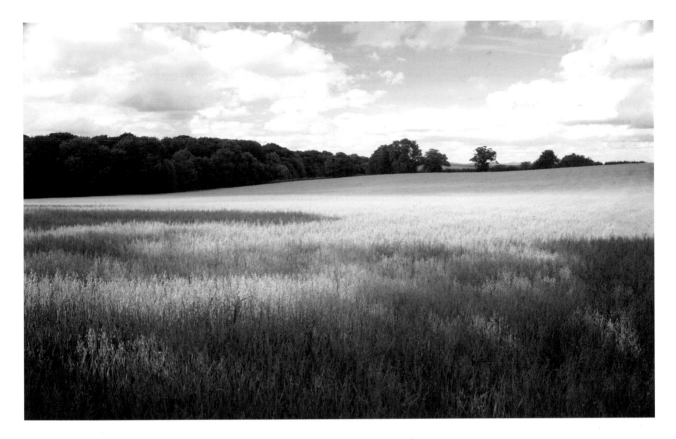

oils). I don't advise using essential oils on eczema as they can increase the irritation.

Great care must be taken to use creams that contain effective preservatives (such as parabens or phenoxyethanol); skin conditions can be made much worse by the bugs found breeding in poorly or unpreserved (usually natural) emollients.

Alternative therapies

There is some evidence for alleviation from hypnotherapy, autogenic training, biofeedback (a technique that helps you monitor and control involuntary physical functions such as breathing, heart rate and muscle contractions) and stress management strategies that calm the mind. Chinese herbal medicine is accepted by some as helpful (although the effect may only be short term). Treatment may involve herbal bath soaks and an extremely bitter tea. Dr David Atherton of The Great Ormond Street Hospital for Children,

Tip

To help babies and small children break the itch-scratch-itch cycle, I like the range of Little Protechtor clothing – which includes a unisex Scratchtite top with built-in Scratch Mitts, made of superfine Cleancool fabric, which contains antibacterial nano-technology silver particles to heal and soothe skin.

www.little-protechtor.com

who is one of the UK's leading paediatric eczema specialists, has been interested in the Chinese herbal approach since the early 1990s, and is particularly impressed by some practitioners' results. Always see a qualified practitioner.

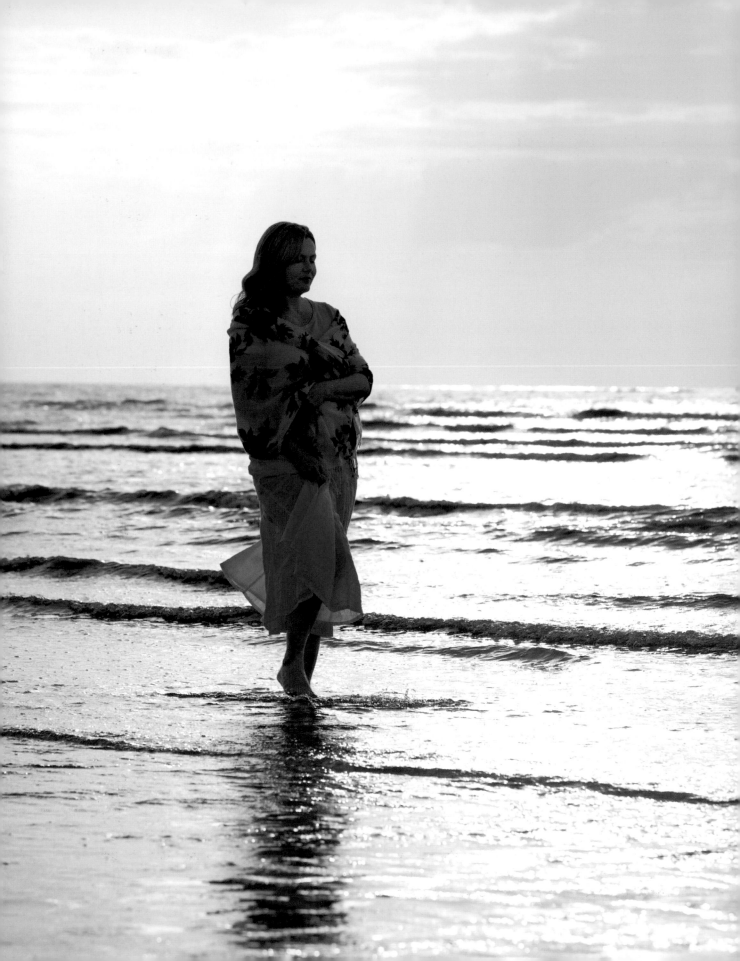

Calming things to do

Relaxing massage, taking exercise, walking in the woods or by the sea, prayer, yoga, meditation, general 'time-out', listening to or taking part in music.

Lifestyle

Dry skin makes the condition worse, so avoid hot baths and showers; wash or bathe quickly to lessen contact with water; use an emollient wash rather than soap; after bathing/showering, apply lubricating cream within three minutes to help trap the moisture in the skin.

Avoid any products containing sodium lauryl or laureth sulfate (soap, detergent, baby wipes, bubble bath, bath gels and even aqueous cream – which may come from a doctor); swap to natural household cleaners that tend not to contain the more harsh synthetic chemicals (such as bio-enzymes) or perfumes.

Choose cotton or silk clothing and bedding, as synthetic fabrics and wool can be irritating.

The droppings of the house dust mite, which thrives in warm damp places such as mattresses and bedding, as well as soft furnishing and carpets, may trigger attacks, so hot-wash bedding weekly and air thoroughly. Consider replacing carpets with wood or tiles. Wash bedding at 60°C weekly and air daily, and do the same with soft toys. (Put non-washable toys in the freezer for 24 hours. You can do this with pillows, too.)

Diet

Follow an anti-inflammatory diet (see chapter 7).

Food allergies may be an important trigger in children with severe atopic eczema: the most common ones are cow's milk, eggs, peanuts, other nuts and kiwi fruit. However, it is very important to seek specialist advice, because it's such a complex area. Avoid high-street allergy testing, advises Professor Michael Cork of the University of Sheffield, as it is of no benefit; 'it takes years of experience to interpret allergy tests,' he says.

A significant number of people with eczema also have an overgrowth of candida in the gut. Cutting out sugars and starches will help restore balance to the gut, and I suggest taking a good probiotic supplement; there is some compelling evidence that probiotic yogurts improve the skin barrier function.

Drink lots of water to help flush toxins out of the body. Six to eight glasses daily is a good habit to aquire.

Contact Dermititis

This inflammatory condition occurs when the skin is irritated by contact with an external substance. There are two types: irritant and allergic.

Irritant contact dermatitis, which accounts for about 80 per cent of cases, occurs when an irritant causes direct injury to the skin, usually on the hands. Common irritants include soaps, detergents and various foodstuffs. Irritants are often job-related; those working in hairdressing, cleaning, building, metal engineering and horticulture commonly experience irritant contact dermatitis, due to the substances they're handling daily. Those with dry skin and/or an atopic condition (eczema, asthma, or hayfever) are more likely to suffer.

Allergic contact dermatitis is due to a 'delayed hypersensitivity' reaction, involving the immune system, where the body first becomes sensitised to a substance, then, at a later stage, allergic to any contact with a particular substance or group of related substances. Any part of the body can be affected. The most common allergens are nickel, rubber, formaldehyde, skin medications (including topical steroid creams), fragrances, hairdressing chemicals and some plants.

The treatment for both types is to track the offending substance and avoid it, if possible, or take protective action, such as wearing rubber gloves (non-latex brands, if you are sensitive to latex). Then treat the eruption in the same way as you would eczema, except that you do not need to use the specific eczema herbs.

Psoriasis

About 1 in 50 people suffer from this distressing condition, which appears as itchy dry red patches, covered with silvery scales. Scratching the patches causes them to crack and become very sore. Overactive T-cells in the immune system set off an inflammatory process that makes skin cells multiply 1,000 times faster than normal.

No one is certain about exactly what causes psoriasis, but there is a genetic link and stress aggravates the condition. As with eczema, poor liver function is a suspect, as is leaky gut syndrome (where toxins in the gut weaken the gut wall and pass into the bloodstream).

Smoking more than 15 cigarettes a day is strongly linked to the development of psoriasis in adults, particularly women; other causal factors are excess alcohol consumption, high dairy intake, obesity, type 2 diabetes and hypothyroidism.

Natural prescription (see pages 186–7)

A good liver cleanser helps to eliminate toxins from the bloodstream that could potentially inflame the skin.

Vitamin A helps to maintain healthy outer skin cells and prevent the silver scales.

Vitamin D in its biologically active form (D3) has been shown to be deficient in people with psoriasis, so for this (and other reasons) it makes sense to supplement diet with this important vitamin.

EFA deficiency (Essential Fatty Acids), which results in pro-inflammatory compounds in the bloodstream, is common among psoriatics, so an EFA supplement is vital. EFAs also help skin health in general. Several studies have shown that fish oil, which contains an EFA called eicosapentanoic acid (somewhat confusingly referred to as EPA), helps alleviate psoriasis in some.

Those with inflammatory skin conditions are often deficient in zinc; it also helps the immune system, as well as encouraging the production of anti-inflammatory compounds in the bloodstream. (Take as zinc picolinate.)

A protein extract made from bovine whey (marketed as Lactoferrin), which has immune regulating and anti-inflammatory effects, has been shown to be helpful in mild to moderate psoriasis.

As with eczema, a combination of herbs including red clover can help clear toxins; see Diet, below.

Emollients are essential to help mend the skin barrier and reduce the scaliness and itchiness. Ceramide-containing emollients such as CeraVe, Mimyx, and Aveeno Eczema Care have shown benefits for psoriasis sufferers. (Ceramides are lipids, or fats, that retain water, regulate cells and repair the skin's barrier; psoriatics have a deficiency of these.)

Topical treatments with plant derivatives are proving effective: these include *Calendula officinalis* aka marigold (see box right), *Aloe vera*, *Berberis aquifolium* (Oregon Grape) capsaicin (from chilli peppers) and curcumin (a compound derived from the spice turmeric).

Natural balms may also help specific patches of irritation, but be wary of essential oils as they can irritate.

Many customers say that Liz Earle Superskin Moisturiser is very helpful for this condition and for mild eczema too.

Diet

* Follow an anti-inflammatory diet (see chapter 7). Avoid fats and sugars, wheat and dairy products, and reduce alcohol consumption.
* Try Dr Stuart's Skin Purify Tea with red clover, nettles and lemon balm, to cleanse body and soothe skin.
* Swedish bitters, an old herbal remedy which stimulates the digestion, is recommended by natural health experts.

Lifestyle

* Reduce stress, or, if that's impossible, at least take steps to manage it.
* Stop smoking: this is vital.

* Sunshine, exercise and sea bathing have been shown to be beneficial. (But patients must take care not to overdo the exposure to UV light.)
* Baths: always bath in cool/warm water, not hot; to loosen scabs, mix in one cup of oatmeal. Also try bathing in Dead Sea Salts, which achieved significant relief in 47 out of 50 patients in a study – maximum improvement came from soaking in 1kg salts, for three baths weekly, over six weeks.

Complementary and alternative therapies

* Individualised homeopathic treatment has been shown to lead to a good response in some patients with chronic skin disease.
* Dead Sea therapy: the minerals in this inland sea have been proven to help patients with psoriasis and the related arthritic condition.
* UVB phototherapy: as with natural sunshine, this light treatment helps persuade cells to slow down and behave more like normal skin; it is effective, but, like sunshine, must be treated with care and should be administered by trained hospital staff.
* PUVA: this light treatment uses UVA light with a plant derivative called a psoralen, which makes the skin more sensitive to light. Like UVB phototherapy, it is a hospital treatment.
* Psychotherapy: emotional upsets are strongly linked to skin flare-ups, particularly in those with psoriasis. Good results have been shown with psychotherapy, hypnotherapy, relaxation techniques and biofeedback.

Marigold (*Calendula*)

The bright orange petals of the pot or English marigold (but not the African marigold or *Tagetes*) have a long history as an excellent remedy for inflamed and angry skin. The compounds identified in Calendula extracts include triterpenoids (including faradiol, glycosides and sapsonins) and herbalists say that these have antiseptic and healing properties which help to prevent the spread of infection and speed up the rate of repair. Research is under way at the University of Strathclyde, Scotland, into the use of a novel marigold compound (christened Van10-4) as a treatment for the scaly plaques of psoriasis, which are notoriously difficult to treat. (Strathclyde Institute of Drug Research has also discovered that certain chemicals in marigold could help heart patients.)

Marigold has been successfully trialled to help treat psoriasis and also leg ulcers

Acne

Acne occurs when pores on the surface of the skin become clogged. Each pore has a follicle, which contains an oil (sebaceous) gland – and, some, a hair. In healthy skin, the oil glands produce the right amount of sebum to help lubricate the skin and dead skin cells are naturally sloughed off the skin surface, then replaced with new ones. In acne, however, the dead skin cells around the follicles do not shed properly, and the result is that the follicles become clogged with whiteheads, which turn into blackheads as they reach the surface and become oxidised, then – if bacteria are present – into spots.

Because the main acne sufferers were teenagers, with boys in the majority, it used to be thought that the cause was an excess of the male hormone testosterone, which stimulates the sebaceous glands to produce more sebum. While this is clearly one trigger, oily skin is not the only trigger and, in fact, African-origin skin, which is very rich in sebum, suffers much less from acne. Increasingly, dermatologists are seeing adults, mainly women, with acne – but, confusingly, they have dry, sensitive skin. As Dr Nicholas Perricone explains in his book *The Acne Prescription*, new wisdom holds that, in this second group, acne begins with inflammation. This occurs at the cellular level, rather than being the result of a blocked pore which comes into contact with bacteria, then becomes inflamed.

When we're stressed or eat poorly, we put our bodies under oxidative stress (see page 14). Our cells then produce pro-inflammatory chemicals called cytokines. One particular cytokine, Interleukin-1, has been shown to the make the skin cells (keratinocytes) sticky. In consequence, dead skin cells don't get exfoliated properly; they build up in the follicle, the pore becomes clogged and infected, and the result is acne.

The solution for both groups of sufferers can be holistic and reflects much of what has been shown to be successful with all sufferers of skin problems.

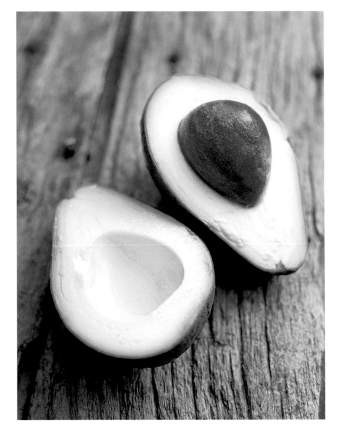

* **Adopt an anti-inflammatory diet (see chapter 7)**
* **Take supplements to control inflammation**
* **Drink plenty of still, pure water**
* **Get 7–8 hours sleep a night**
* **Minimise stress and learn how to control what you can't avoid**
* **Treat existing acne lesions with anti-inflammatory topical creams/lotions**
* **Conventional medication may be useful in the short term for severe cases and can prevent scarring**

Natural prescription (see pages 186–7)

Taking vitamins A and D, and zinc often helps acne sufferers by stimulating healthy new cells. Zinc (choose zinc picolinate, which is well absorbed by the body) heals skin tissue and has hormone-modulating properties.

Omega-3 Essential Fatty Acids balance the inflammatory agent prostaglandin 2, and help with other functions.

Many acne sufferers in their teens and twenties have benefited from using a safe and effective Ayurvedic supplement called Tejaswini, which contains herbs that are believed to cleanse the bloodstream of the hormone metabolites of testosterone.

A topical cream (ActivClear), which contains tea tree, vitamin A and extracts of the herb tribulus, helps to reduce sebum production wherever it is applied.

Diet

To keep blood sugar stable (which helps prevent an inflammatory response), eat three small meals and two snacks a day.

Eat a low-GI diet (see chapter 7), with oily fish and other protein (eg, chicken, turkey, soy products and occasionally beef) at every main meal, plus fresh vegetables, salads and fruit, chopped nuts and ground flaxseeds, yogurt and olive oil. Avocados are a good source of beneficial nutrients.

Antioxidants are also anti-inflammatory, according to Dr Nicholas Perricone, since oxidative stress is one key cause of inflammation. So, in addition to your antioxidant-rich veg and fruit, that means you can eat a little, very dark chocolate (aim for 85 per cent cocoa solids), as chocolate is very high in antioxidants.

Try green tea or chicory, instead of coffee, to maintain stable blood sugar levels and help prevent the inflammatory cascade.

Cutting out cow's milk – substituting soy, almond, oat or rice milk – may help acne sufferers. It's thought that the pregnancy and growth-enhancing hormones in milk – which comes mostly from cows that are simultaneously lactating and pregnant – may affect some people. Skimmed milk seems to cause the most problems; drinking organic milk isn't likely to make a difference, as it still comes from lactating and pregnant cows.

Lifestyle

Meditation, yoga and prayer all reduce stress.

Complementary and alternative therapies

Although specific research data is very limited, a study of acne patients showed that they tended to value CAM (eg, homeopathy, naturopathy, western herbalism and reflexology) over orthodox therapies, because they thought it was more effective, had fewer side effects (drugs such as the contraceptive pill Dianette and Roaccutane have been linked to severe depression and suicidal thoughts) and they had a greater sense of control, which all helped them feel less anxious about their condition.

I would always suggest trying natural therapies first, but acne scarring can be lifelong – and the psychological damage can be profound – so some people may need to take prescribed medication to get it under control.

Open pores

Pores are the opening at the top of follicles. The size of the pore depends mainly on how dilated the follicle is; if it's clogged with dead skin cells and sebum, the follicle will be comparatively fat, and so will the pore. A nice clean narrow follicle will lead into a normal-sized pore. The received wisdom is that if you have open or large pores, you can't change them… But, certainly, applying ice cubes – or some people swear by cucumber juice or skin tonic – can help, on a temporary basis. And I've heard several say that their previously large pores have closed over time with the application of clay-based masks. Interestingly, several women with large pores gave up moisturiser and found the problem got worse; when they re-started, their open pores significantly improved.

Rosacea

The flushing and redness caused by this chronic facial skin condition is really distressing to sufferers – increasingly, young women. Secondary symptoms include facial burning, stinging, papules/pustules, dryness or oiliness. The areas most commonly affected are the cheeks, nose, forehead and chin, but the eyes may be involved too (ocular rosacea), making them sting and feel gritty. Sometimes the skin swells and thickens; if this happens around the nose, it's called rhinopyma, or bulbous nose. (Incidentally, although it's sometimes called acne rosacea, this condition has nothing to do with acne.)

Conventional drug treatment focuses on treating the secondary symptoms, rather than the flushing, now generally believed to be caused by a disorder of the blood vessels in the face, which become hypersensitive to internal and external triggers. This results in more blood flow through the facial skin, causing more inflammation and more damage, making the condition progressively worse. However, no one knows the underlying cause of rosacea, and it is difficult to treat. Some doctors believe that the only effective way of treating the disorder in the blood vessels is to 'shut them off' with laser treatment, used in conjunction with lifestyle changes and skin-calming products. But, even if this does work, it is unlikely to be a permanent cure and may need to be repeated one to three years after the first series of treatments.

There is a wide range of triggers, including alcohol, spicy foods and hot drinks, food intolerances, sunlight and extreme temperatures (such as those found in saunas), stress, anger or embarrassment and excessive exercising.

Research shows that people with rosacea may not produce enough stomach acid (HCl), which helps digestion, and that supplementing diet with this at mealtimes can improve symptoms. Additionally, stress often interferes with HCl production, and many sufferers experience much worse symptoms when stressed. One study found that members of a subgroup who had indigestion after eating fatty foods were deficient in the pancreatic enzyme lipase, which helps to digest fat. When they were given pancreatic enzyme supplements with meals, their indigestion and rosacea improved. Constipation may be a contributing factor, too.

Drugs that cause blood vessels to dilate are another risk factor, and a small skin mite (*Demodex folliculorum*) occurs in far greater numbers on the faces of rosacea sufferers and may be an exacerbating factor, stimulating an immune response that results in inflammation.

Reproductive hormones may be involved, too. Many women report more flushing episodes and increased numbers of bumps and pimples at the mid-month point in their cycle and during menopause.

So, rosacea is complicated. Leaving aside laser

Milia

Milia are tiny white bumps or small cysts which appear when dead skin becomes trapped in little pockets on the skin surface. Primary milia are found on the faces of babies and adults, while secondary milia occur in areas of inflamed or injured skin, particularly sun-damaged skin. In babies, they tend to disappear within the first few weeks of life. In adults, however, they are difficult to remove without the risk of scarring, so it is best to consult your doctor or dermatologist. (Some skilled beauty therapists are adept at dealing with them with a fine needle and magnifying mirror.) The most likely risk is smothering the skin with heavy skincare products, which prevent dead skin cells being exfoliated. So avoid anything with mineral oil – which can clog pores – exfoliate regularly and opt for light, simple products. If you get milia around your eyes, or on the lids, you may need to change your eye make-up and remover.

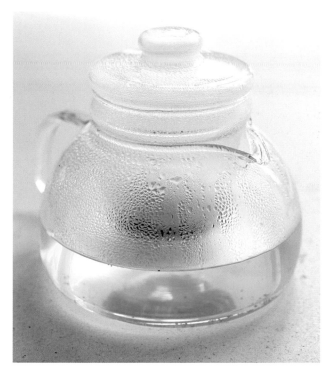

Thread veins

Thread veins (spider, broken or capillary veins) are small dilated veins or capillaries (blood vessels) found on the cheek, nose and legs. They are usually red, though larger veins may appear to be bluey purple. They can start to show up as a result of sun exposure, smoking, thinning of the skin due to over-use of steroidal creams, and often after pregnancy or weight increase. Conventional treatments include laser therapy and sclerotherapy (saline injections) but there are some good alternative treatments and supplements. Topical treatments containing horse chestnut (which is said to increase local circulation and tonify capillaries) may help; pycnogenol (which is said to strengthen the capillary network) and witch hazel (which may help to shrink the capillaries). Supplementing with dietary pycnogenol could help.

treatment (which may be effective, but is expensive), it makes sense to start by identifying individual triggers and avoiding them as much as possible. After that, it's a case of following an anti-inflammatory regime in much the same way as for acne, including diet, stress management, supplements and soothing topical products.

Natural prescription (see pages 186–7)

Essential Fatty Acids are the best starting point for supplements, because they have an anti-inflammatory effect, help to cleanse the colon (thus improving any problems with the gut) and also help to balance hormones. In a small study, a comprehensive fatty acid supplement containing omega-3, 6 and 9 (Ultimate Beauty Oil, by Viridian) significantly helped some participants.

A good probiotic will help balance bacteria in the gut, which are known to have an effect on the skin and help get rid of acids and toxins that may kick off inflammation.

Topical treatments containing specific compounds have been shown to help rosacea in clinical trials. These include creams or ointments containing one or more of

Chrysanthellum indicum, green tea, liquorice and niacinamide, a form of vitamin B3 (nb: don't be tempted to take this as a supplement internally).

Azelaic acid cream, which is based on derivatives of wheat, rye and barley, appears to be as effective as topical metronidazole (an antibiotic) at reducing papules/pustules and slightly better at reducing skin redness. Physicians rated the overall improvement with azelaic acid as better than with metronidazole and patients preferred it, although some experienced stinging on application. ActivClear cream contains a combination of skin-repairing and soothing agents, including tea tree oil, zinc sulphate, vitamins A, B1, B5, B6 and E, plus the herb tribulus, a yellow-flowered plant also known as puncture vine. Pycnogenol, an extract from the marine pine bark tree, has a powerful anti-inflammatory effect, and may help the fragile capillaries and strengthen outer layers of the skin. A cream containing MSM, a form of sulphur (which is antibacterial and anti-inflammatory), aloe vera and calendula is popular with some sufferers.

A good mineral-based sunscreen is vital, as UV light and heat will aggravate the condition, as will cold winds.

Dark circles

Most people get dark circles under their eyes – or even all round the eye area – at some point.

Surprisingly, the most common cause isn't lack of sleep (although it does have an effect) but nasal congestion. The main reason for dark circles on pale skin tones is being able to see blood vessels under the skin. When your nose is bunged up, veins that usually drain from your eyes into your nose become dilated and darker. Fluid retention can also cause the capillaries under the eyes to become dilated and contribute to the same effect. Conditions that cause fluid retention (such as heart, thyroid, kidney and liver diseases) or medications that cause blood vessel dilation may be a factor (always discuss it with your doctor). Dark circles may also be a sign of dehydration. In those with darker skin tones, dark circles are sometimes, unfortunately, genetic.

Ageing can provoke the appearance of dark circles, because the skin becomes thinner (and may be paler) so the blood vessels show up more: sun damage contributes, because it weakens the skin.

Rubbing itchy eyes, due to allergies and hayfever, can also result in dark circles; hayfever sufferers often notice them at the height of the season.

Another cause often overlooked is overproduction of the pigment melanin in the eye area. This may be because the very thin skin there is more sensitive to the sun. Sun damage will also thin skin further, by degrading collagen. Wearing sunscreen and big sunglasses can help with the problem, and prevent more pigmentation and skin thinning.

Iron-deficiency anaemia results in less oxygen passing through the bloodstream, which produces a bluish tint. It's important to have a blood test, to make sure anaemia is not the cause. If it is, take a non-constipating, highly absorbable form of iron, such as the product Iron Bisglycinate, by HealthAid. (The ferrous iron formulas prescribed for this by most doctors often result in nausea and constipation, according to Dr Ivor Cavill, senior lecturer in dermatology at Cardiff University School of Medicine.)

Natural prescription (see pages 186–7)

Supplements containing vitamin C, or grapeseed extract, or pycnogenol contain antioxidant compounds that may help to strengthen blood vessels. (Anyone on blood-thinning medication, such as Warfarin, should take these only under medical supervision.)

Topical creams containing vitamin K may help. Other ingredients in 'topicals' include eyebright, horse chestnut, gingko and yarrow, which increase localised circulation – also witch hazel, for its astringent properties, which may help to shrink the capillaries. Pycnogenol and green tea may also help strengthen the tissue in the eye area.

Lifestyle

Be sure to get enough sleep and STOP SMOKING!

Quick fixes

A cold compress will help constrict blood vessels and normalise tissue colour: wring out a flannel in very cold water, place on eyes and lie down for 10–15 minutes as many times as possible. Alternatively, smooth an ice cube – in a cotton hanky or muslin cloth – round the eye area, which also reduces puffiness. Lie down with chilled cucumber slices, or slices of raw potato, or plain teabags (rich in natural tannins) over your eyes.

Complementary and alternative medicine

Traditional Chinese Medicine (TCM) holds that a bluish cast under the eyes is due to an imbalance in kidney energy (the under-eye area is linked to the kidneys in TCM): if you decide to consult a TCM practitioner, always choose someone who is registered and appropriately qualified.

Diet

Feast on cranberries, blueberries and bilberries, blackcurrants, onions and legumes, garnished with lots of parsley and washed down with green tea (or black); they contain the antioxidants that may help to fortify blood vessels. Drink plenty of water to combat dehydration, flush out toxins and discourage fluid retention (if you don't drink enough water, your body will want to retain it, resulting in fluid retention and toxins staying in the system). Cut down on dietary salt, which may contribute to dilated blood vessels.

Hair and scalp problems

'Shoulder snow', as dandruff is euphemistically known, is the excessive shedding of the cells on the scalp. Dead skin is shed constantly from our bodies as cells renew themselves and our scalp sheds more than any other part. Normally, skin cells mature in about a month and are shed gradually, so the process is virtually unnoticeable. With dandruff, cell turnover speeds up and cells are being shed on a weekly – even daily – basis.

But, rest assured that, far from being the social outcast condition portrayed in advertisements, dandruff is one that most people suffer from at some point in their lives.

There are three main causes:
* The most common dandruff, which affects 75 per cent of people during their life, is pityriasis capitis (which means 'scaly head'). It's caused by a minute yeast-like fungus called Pityrosporum ovale (also known as malassezia). People with dandruff have higher amounts of pityrosporum than usual; they often have a history of childhood eczema. The flakes seem dry and the scalp is dry and itchy. It's rare in children but increases in the teens and twenties.
* Left untreated, common dandruff can lead to seborrheic dermatitis, an inflammatory disorder where the outermost layer of the skin peels off excessively, producing flakes. Both the hair and scales seem greasy, and there are patches of red, scaly, itchy skin, which may also occur on the face, chest and other parts of the body. Flare-ups can be triggered by stress or illness.
* Scalp psoriasis is often very localised, around the ears and the back of the head, although it may be dotted all over. The scales are quite thick and red; the redness may also be seen round the hairline. Many patients experience severe itching and a feeling of tightness or soreness.

Psoriasis is known as 'the waxing and waning condition', so it may go away or only flare up occasionally. GPs can prescribe a coal tar de-scaling agent such as cocois, or a scalp ointment combining coconut oil, coal tar solution, sulphur and salicylic acid.

Here is a suggested course of action:
* Those with very dry hair and skin should eat plenty of oily fish or consider a fish oil supplement. Biotin deficiency has been linked to seborrheic dermatitis, so you could try taking this either on its own or as part of a B complex supplement.
* If you work in a very dehydrating environment, such as an aircraft, take care to drink lots of water and use moisturising products on hair and skin. If you work in an air-conditioned office, try putting bowls of water around your desk or buy a small humidifier.
* If you can see any red patches, visit your GP or consult a qualified trichologist.
* Don't scratch your scalp: it will make the condition worse, and may break the skin, leaving it vulnerable to bacterial infection.
* Double the frequency of washing your hair (unless you already do it every day): British trichologist Dr Hugh Rushton says the cause of the snowstorm may simply be an accumulation of dead skin cells, due to not washing your hair often enough. Take time to gently agitate your scalp all over and rinse thoroughly until you can't feel any shampoo left. Follow with a conditioner if you wish. Do this for a month.
* Plant extracts to look for in shampoos include chamomile, red clover, echinacea and nettle to calm the inflammation on the scalp and red cedar oil (thuja) to help

control fungi (not for children or the sensitive-skinned).

* I suggest avoiding sodium lauryl or laureth sulfate in shampoos, as I have found they make flaky scalps worse.

* If your scalp is still flaking after four weeks, try any anti-dandruff shampoo to combat the fungus. Use this consistently for another month. If the condition doesn't improve, then go to your family doctor.

* Avoid using products such as hair spray, volumising mousse, styling sprays or relaxing preparations, which can leave a residue that looks like dandruff, as well as exacerbating an already dry scalp.

* Consider giving up dairy products for a month to see if it makes a difference. It won't help everyone, but some patients with an eczematous type of dandruff improve with this simple dietary shift.

Lemon balm has antiviral properties which help to heal cold sores quickly

Warts and cold sores

A wart is a small, rough, raised lump, caused by a viral infection. There are many different types, varying in shape and site of infection, ranging from the common wart (*verruca vulgaris*) to genital warts. They can be highly contagious, so never share towels and always wear something on your feet at gyms or swimming pools. Many patients have found this regime (devised by pharmacist Shabir Daya) effective for common warts (but don't try it for other types, especially genital warts). Take lysine daily on an empty stomach; this inhibits viral replication by blocking the uptake of arginine, a major 'food source' for the virus, which it needs in order to multiply. Also take a good immune enhancer, such as astragalus, to help eradicate the virus more quickly from the body. Topically, use a 'paint' with manuka honey and the herb horopito from New Zealand, applied twice a day to the warts. Manuka (*Leptospermum scoparium*) is known for its germicidal properties and the 65million-year-old horopito (*Pseudowintera colorata*) for its antifungal and antiviral properties.

Cold sores are clusters of small, painful, unsightly blisters on the lip and around the mouth and, like warts, are caused by a virus. In this case, it's the herpes simplex virus. This virus also needs arginine to replicate, so it's wise to take a supplement of lysine, as above.

Topically, research shows that *Melissa officinalis* or lemon balm calms the inflammation and itching, as well as having antiviral properties which help to heal the sore quickly. Make your own remedy by mixing a drop of pure melissa essential oil with a teaspoon of grapeseed or almond oil and apply with a cotton bud at the first sign of tingling (or try Liz Earle Spot On, which contains melissa oil).

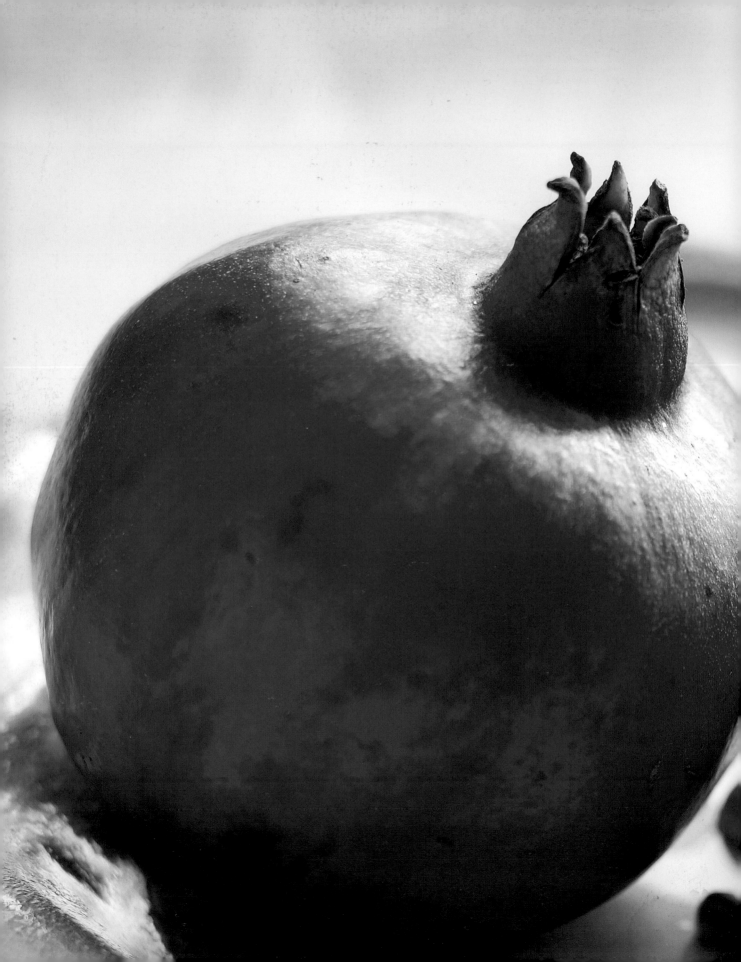

Chapter Seven

FEED YOUR SKIN

It's no surprise that the skin, our largest organ, responds to what we eat. So, keeping it nourished is a must if we want radiant glowing skin – and the good news is that the whole body benefits too.

Feed your skin

Good food gives us the building blocks for good skin. Here are some of my secrets for eating well – for your health and your skin.

Food has been a focus for me for many years. I've written about it, campaigned for meaningful food labelling and taken a public stand against the genetic modification of our basic foods. Nowadays I feel even more passionate – if that's possible – about eating well and all the many issues surrounding it.

I started writing books when I was pregnant with my first child, Lily, now in her late teens. I knew that what I put in my shopping trolley was creating a new life inside me and that the ultimate responsibility for nourishing my baby rested solely on my shoulders. I became convinced of the arguments for producing food organically, not only because shunning pesticides, fertilisers and GM technology is better for the planet, but also because the food contains fewer traces of toxic chemical residues and tends to be more nutritious. After years living in London, my husband and I plunged head first into commercial food production and we now live on an organic farm, rearing traditional and rare-breed sheep, pigs and chickens. We also have an organic kitchen garden and grow a few herbs and botanicals for good measure.

Even in London, I discovered that you really don't need much space to grow your own. Leading UK organic herb grower, Jekka McVicar, suggests planting a delicious mixed-leaf 'cut and come again' salad crop in a simple 1-litre plant pot. I grew salad leaves, edible flowers such as nasturtiums, and herbs in a window box. (One couple went much further and were completely self-sufficient in veggies from a small rooftop garden.) I also ordered a weekly organic fruit and veg box, with a variety of seasonal produce delivered to the door.

As a mother of four I'm also determined to teach my brood how to cook good food – it tastes better, is more nutritious and can be done on a small budget. Pre-packaged food is often devoid of flavour, costs significantly more and creates much more packaging waste. Despite this, cooking is a skill we have lost from the many school curriculums, so few young people know how to cook even simple foods. The irony is that most children and teenagers love to cook. My local family doctor bought her 15-year-old son a cookery book with an explanatory DVD. It was so successful that, during the school holidays, she returned from her practice each day to a delicious, home-cooked supper ready to serve.

Eating together round a table is so important, both for catching up and eating a proper meal – slowly. We aim to sit down as a family once a day – more often at weekends and during the holidays. I ban eating while standing up, reading or watching television. Food is not simply a substance for shovelling in unawares; it is for savouring and valuing – even if it's just a 15-minute lunchtime snack. Eating slowly is important for the digestive juices too, as the anticipatory salivation releases digestive enzymes that make food easier to digest and absorb. Try putting down your fork after each mouthful and chewing twenty times before swallowing (the famed Mayr Clinic advocate 40 times). This helps to release more nutrients from food, makes it easier to digest and avoids overeating, by making you feel fuller, sooner. It also means we eat less, as it takes about 20 minutes for the signals of satiety to reach our brain. Eating little and often suits most people far better than devouring three (or, all too often, one) big meals a day.

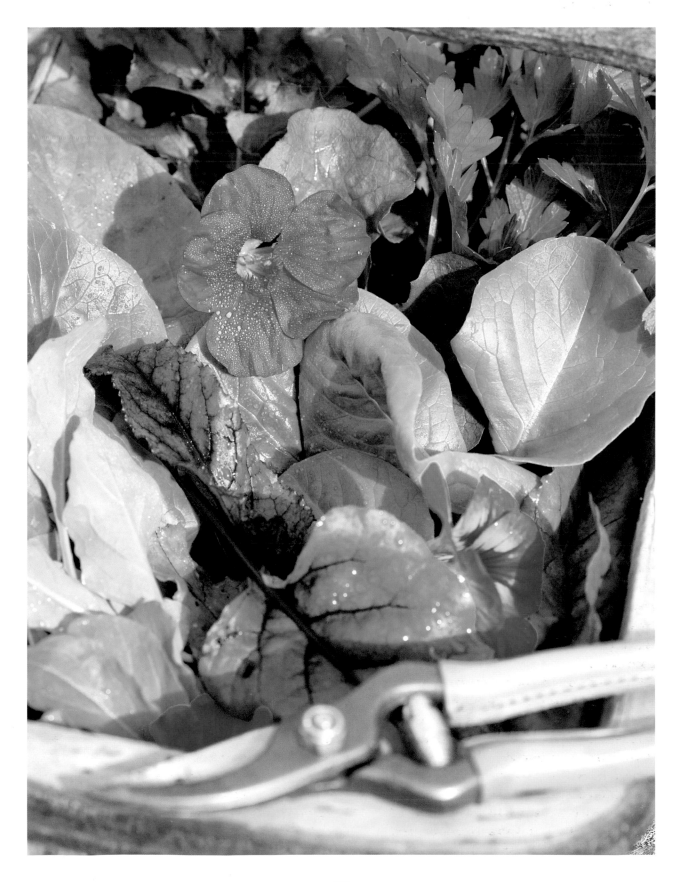

Foods we should love or leave – and why

We really are what we eat. Nowadays we know the complex truth that underlies this adage. Everything that we consume is processed by the body in some way and goes towards making either good – or bad – components. Nowhere do the results of this process show more obviously than in our skin.

According to the old nursery rhyme, little girls are made of sugar and spice and all things nice. While I'm quite happy to believe the last bit, sugar is a different matter. In fact, skin is made up of water (about 70 per cent), protein (about 25 per cent) and lipids, or fats (about 2 per cent) with various chemicals making up the remainder. Sugar is a real skin foe, but more of that later.

Protein is indispensable to healthy skin, hair and nails, as well as to blood cells, the immune and nervous systems and enzymes, which make reactions occur. In other words, everything! To be accurate, it's the amino acids in proteins that are the building blocks of the body. When we eat foods containing proteins, our digestive system breaks down the protein into its component amino acids, and joins them together again as the structural proteins we need. There are 20 amino acids, 11 of which our body can make, but the other 9 must come from our food.

Although technically we could obtain all the nutrients we need from plant sources, the so-called 'complete proteins', which contain all the 'essential amino acids' our body needs, come mainly from animal sources (meat, game, fish, dairy and eggs). Ensuring you get the necessary nutrients from a vegetarian or vegan diet is much more complicated, particularly for Westerners who, unlike say the Jains in India, do not have a long tradition of eating in this way. In fact, the only plant source that contains all the essential amino acids is soy and its derivatives, such as

tofu (I recommend choosing GM-free varieties).

For proteins to do their job effectively, they need Essential Fatty Acids (EFAs) plus a good spread of vitamins and minerals. The body can't make EFAs, so they, too, must come from the diet: find them in oily fish (mackerel, herring, tuna, salmon, sardines, anchovies), eggs, flaxseeds, flaxseed and rapeseed oil, walnuts and dark green vegetables. Vitamins and minerals come from protein and dairy, and in abundance from vegetables and fruit. Vegetables also contain crucial fibre to keep the elimination system working well, ridding the body of toxins that could impair our health and skin.

Then there's water: dehydration is known to be a major problem for your entire body, including the brain. Some scientists say that drinking any type of liquid (milk, tea, coffee) is as good as drinking water: my own experience is that I feel and look much better if I drink lots of still, pure water. Naturopath, Roderick Lane, maintains that when you consume liquids other than water, which inevitably contain other chemical constituents, the body perceives them as food. This uses up more energy (which could be better employed) and takes longer for the body to absorb. So, the drill for me and my family is to sip 6–8 large glasses of water a day, mostly between meals. Flavour with fresh lemon, cucumber sticks or fresh root ginger to ring the changes. Keep a bottle of water with you when you go out.

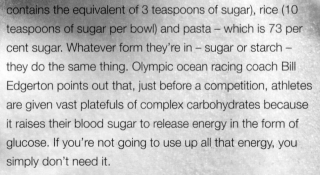

Sugar

Yes, it makes us pile on the pounds, but that may be the least of the damage. As I discussed in Chapter 6, scientists now know that anything that causes a rise in blood sugar levels causes inflammation. Although inflammation is a natural healing reaction, it can easily get out of control or be triggered inadvertently and many researchers say that it is proving to be the basis of virtually every disease process from cancer, heart disease, joint problems and dementia to skin problems (such as acne and eczema) and skin ageing.

The problem occurs when we have too much sugar in our body: the sugar molecules attach themselves to proteins (remember, those are the basic structure of skin, blood vessels, cartilage and many other parts of the body). Known as glycosylation (or glycation), this process causes not only hardening of the arteries and stiff joints, but – when the sugar clings to collagen, degrading this protein which is vital for skin tone and 'bounceback' – wrinkles and sags. A build up of excess sugar also affects the antioxidant proteins in the body, which protect against free radical formation, leaving us vulnerable to cell damage and more visible skin ageing.

Lack of sleep is also implicated here, because when we're sleep-deprived, levels of a hormone called cortisol rise, pushing up blood sugar, so stimulating the release of insulin, which sends sugar to the cells – and, to complete the vicious circle, triggers a craving for sugar.

One very important thing to take on board: sugar is not just the white stuff we put in our tea and find in sweets, cakes, biscuits, puddings and so on. It's also in fruit – that's fructose. Starch and sugar are the two main types of carbohydrates, and both of them, once digested, become sugar in your body. So you will also be eating sugar when you eat grains in the shape of bread (1 slice of white bread contains the equivalent of 3 teaspoons of sugar), rice (10 teaspoons of sugar per bowl) and pasta – which is 73 per cent sugar. Whatever form they're in – sugar or starch – they do the same thing. Olympic ocean racing coach Bill Edgerton points out that, just before a competition, athletes are given vast platefuls of complex carbohydrates because it raises their blood sugar to release energy in the form of glucose. If you're not going to use up all that energy, you simply don't need it.

Vegetables do contain carbohydrates but this 'dietary fibre' can't be digested, so it doesn't turn to sugar, except in the case of root veg such as potatoes and parsnips.

Also, try not to consume foods with artificial sweeteners such as aspartame and saccharin, which have been shown to increase appetite (so not much good for dieters), may lead to hyperactivity and depression, and can be addictive. At home, we use xylitol, a natural sweetener, which reduces tooth decay and supports bones.

Green beauty

Fresh fruits and vegetables,
together with top-quality protein,
are great allies for radiant skin.

I believe the best way to eat – and certainly the way that suits me and my family – is along the lines of low-GL (glycaemic load). Dr Mabel Blades, a leading nutritionist and dietitian says, 'The GL has an important influence on health as it takes into account the amount of carbohydrate in a food plus the Glycaemic Index (GI) and therefore has a powerful effect on blood sugar levels. Keeping blood sugar levels stable means that not only do you feel better, but it also stops the longing for a sugar high and snacks high in fat when the blood sugar plummets.' This table, provided by Dr Blades, gives you the GL index of everyday foods as well as their calorie content. Foods are rated according to whether they are low (0-10), medium (11-19) or high (20+) GL. These figures are intended for guidance only, but give a good indication of what to look out for.

A benefit of the GL diet for me is hugely increased energy. Like most people, I can easily slump into lethargy and fatigue if I eat poorly. By stabilising blood sugar, and thus insulin production, it keeps my weight pretty constant. This way of eating is also proving very effective for people with raised cholesterol and triglycerides, as well as those at risk of diabetes, by stabilising insulin production. It can all seem a bit complicated, but if you stick to the food friends I suggest you will be doing well.

Try to eat breakfast, lunch and dinner, with (healthy) snacks mid-morning and afternoon, and last thing at night. Never leave more than 3 hours between eating – your blood sugar starts waning between 2–3 hours after eating. If you eat when blood sugar is low, you are more likely to stuff in lots of sugary/starchy foods, which will give you a quick high – and an equally quick low, because raising blood sugar rapidly stimulates insulin, which moves sugar out of the cells, so creating a 'vacancy' which your body wants to fill immediately.

Interestingly, cooking and processing food can soften and refine it, resulting in a higher GI as the food is digested more rapidly and quickly raises the blood sugar level. Help to slow down your digestion by eating foods that are minimally processed, include the original seeds/husks (for grains), are chunky rather than puréed and lightly cooked (so eat your vegetables crunchy and your pasta al dente!).

The Glycaemic Load table

FOOD	PORTION SIZE	KCAL	GL INDEX
Fruits			
Apple	medium	47	4
Apricots, dried	one	19	1
Avocado	small	190	0
Banana	medium	95	12
Cranberry juice	wine glass	61	8
Grapefruit	half	30	2
Grapes red/white	10	30	4
Melon	small slice	28	4
Vegetables			
Broccoli, boiled	1 spear	12	0+
Cauliflower, boiled	medium	28	0
Courgette, cooked	medium	19	0+
Tomatoes	1 cherry	3	0
Meat and Poultry			
Beef mince extra lean	100g	225	0
Chicken leg, raw	100g	193	0
Lamb lean, raw	100g	153	0
Pork diced lean, raw	100g	122	0
Fish			
Cod, raw	150g	120	0
Mackerel, smoked	100g	354	0
Salmon, fresh	150g	270	0
Prawns, raw	100g	76	0
Eggs and Dairy, including soya alternatives			
Egg, raw	average egg	75	0
Cheddar	25g	104	0
Milk, semi-skimmed	100ml	46	1
Milk, soya	100ml	32	1
Yogurt, fat-free, plain	150g pot	81	3
Fats and Oils			
Butter	medium spread	74	0
Olive oil	1 tablespoon	98	0
Starchy Carbohydrates, Pulses and Nuts			
Dark chocolate	25g	127	6.5
Milk chocolate	25g	130	7
Honey	10g	29	5
Sugar (sucrose)	10g	39	7
Granary Bread	thick slice	83	8
White bread	thick slice	82	10
Porridge with water	bowl	46	3
Pasta, boiled	average portion	129	13
Basmati rice, boiled	small portion	138	18
Brown rice, boiled	small portion	141	22
White rice, boiled	small portion	138	30
Potato, boiled	2 egg size	72	17
Soya beans, cooked	3 tablespoons	141	1
Lentils, boiled	3 tablespoons	103	5
Peanuts, dry roasted	100g	589	1

Food friends

Protein

Try to include a little protein in every main meal (one egg, 40-70g organic or free-range poultry, meat or oily fish, a small tub of yogurt or cottage cheese, or 100ml milk – try goats' and sheep's cheese and yogurt for variety or if you are sensitive to cow's milk). And don't forget about nuts and seeds (walnuts, almonds, brazil nuts; flax, sunflower and pumpkin seeds, flaxseed and rapeseed oil). Don't grill meat or fish until blackened, because that triggers damaging free radicals in the food.

Fruits and vegetables

Aim to eat five to seven portions daily (each the amount you can fit on your palm), in a rainbow of colours. Spinach, watercress, spirulina and (dried) seaweed contain useful amounts of omega-3. Eat fruit between meals, if possible, or at the beginning, but not at the end: the sugars ferment in your gut, 'trapped' by preceding food that is slower to be digested, causing bloating and other problems. But cut down on root vegetables – particularly potatoes and parsnips – because they contain so many starches.

Good fats

Fats are essential for the functioning of our whole body, including the brain. We also need fats to absorb fat-soluble vitamins (A, D, E and K). However, all fats are not born equal! Some are very good for you (Essential Fatty Acids, which I have written about extensively for topical application), and some harmful (mainly saturated and hydrogenated transfats).

Essential Fatty Acids (EFAs) are divided into two main groups: omega-3 and omega-6. It's also essential to consume these in the right ratio: which is 2:1 of omega-6 to omega-3. Experts agree that many diseases today, including heart disease, stem from the proportion shooting up to 9:1, or even more, mainly due to the large amounts of corn and sunflower oil in the typical Western diet.

To get plenty of omega-3, eat oily fish, egg yolk, nuts, nut oils and flaxseed. Cold-pressed rapeseed oil is also a useful source. Omega-6 is found in egg yolk, seeds and seed oils (sunflower, safflower and sesame), whole grains, and some vegetables. Also in evening primrose and borage oil. In practice, if you try to eat plenty of omega-3 rich fish and cut down – or preferably cut out – processed foods and corn and sunflower oils, you will be consuming about the right ratio. 'Good' fats also include olive oil – I cook with ordinary 'pure' olive oil, as it has a lighter taste than extra virgin, which I only use in salad dressings and sauces.

Fresh juices

It's expensive to buy these, so I tend to squeeze one or two oranges and savour a few mouthfuls of deliciously fresh juice instead of swigging cartons of the pasteurised stuff. (Remember to sip through a straw to save your tooth enamel – particularly important for children.) At weekends, I use my electric juicer to make fresh apple, carrot and ginger juice. Simply chop 4 apples, 1 large carrot (topped and tailed but not peeled) and a peeled 2cm chunk of fresh ginger and pop through the machine, then sip slowly.

Good grains

The key here is to eat less rather than none at all (unless you are really trying to lose weight, in which case limit yourself to 60g daily), and to eat non-refined varieties. Look for organic oats, wholegrain bread (or rye or spelt) made the old-fashioned way, so it rises overnight and is much easier on the digestion, brown rice, wholemeal pasta, plus the ancient grains including quinoa, kamut, spelt and faro. So try not to eat processed foods like certain breads, pies, pizza, cakes, biscuits, candy/cereal bars or other refined carbohydrates containing white sugar and/or white flour.

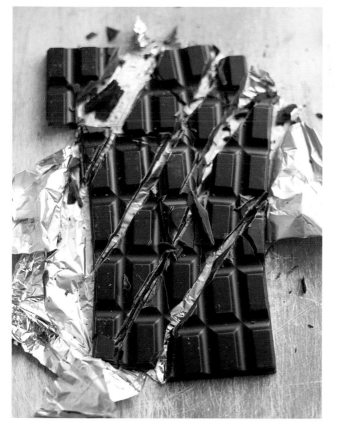

Chocolate

I bring good news for chocolate lovers (like me): eat a little of the darkest chocolate you can – with a minimum of 70 per cent cocoa solids – and it's really good for you. The real McCoy helps diminish appetite, prevents the cravings of commercial chocolate, is the highest food source of magnesium and is very high in antioxidants. These include catechins and phenols, more frequently highlighted in black tea. Dark chocolate contains four times as many catechins as black tea and its phenols help prevent free-radical cell damage. In fact, good milk chocolate (such as Green & Black's) contains 34 per cent cocoa solids – a mixture of cocoa mass and cocoa butter (which is more than many types of mass-market plain dark chocolate). 'Junk choc', on the other hand, is full of sugar, and guaranteed to send your blood sugar rocketing up, then plunging down again.

More cocoa solids means less room for unhealthy fillers, such as hydrogenated (hardened) vegetable oils – aka trans-fats – and sugar, so, the higher the percentage of cocoa solids, the better the chocolate is for us.

Mass-market chocolate tends to contain about 20 per cent cocoa solids and some brands may have as little as 7 per cent, with high levels of vegetable oils instead. In consequence, the EU has suggested that some British brands be re-named 'vegolate' as their low cocoa content means they shouldn't really be called chocolate at all! Plain chocolate is a low-GI food, as it contains so little sugar; you can buy sugar-free raw chocolate, but it doesn't taste that fabulous, so my advice is to eat small amounts of the best-quality dark chocolate you can – let each square melt on your tongue to get the full taste sensation.

Nuts and seeds

These are the life force of plants, absolutely bursting with nutrients, including protein (so very good for vegetarians), EFAs, vitamins (notably, skin-friendly vitamin E) and minerals; and they are high in fibre.

Make a trail mix to take with you as a snack (see page 154). I also prefer nut butters instead of peanut butter (actually a legume); my favourites are almond and hazelnut. I also like mixed-seed butters, made with sunflower, sesame and pumpkin seeds. They're great for a quick breakfast snack, by the spoonful straight from the container, with oatcakes or toast (rye bread is wonderful). Sprinkle a mixture of nuts and seeds on salads, muesli and porridge.

For salads, try adding deliciously crunchy sprouted seeds; buy them ready-sprouted, or make your own – you will find kits at most health-food stores.

Treat

Almonds are a rich source of vegetable protein: for maximum bio-availability (absorption), Ayurvedic experts suggest soaking in room temperature water for 12–24 hours, then peel and eat 6 or 7 daily.

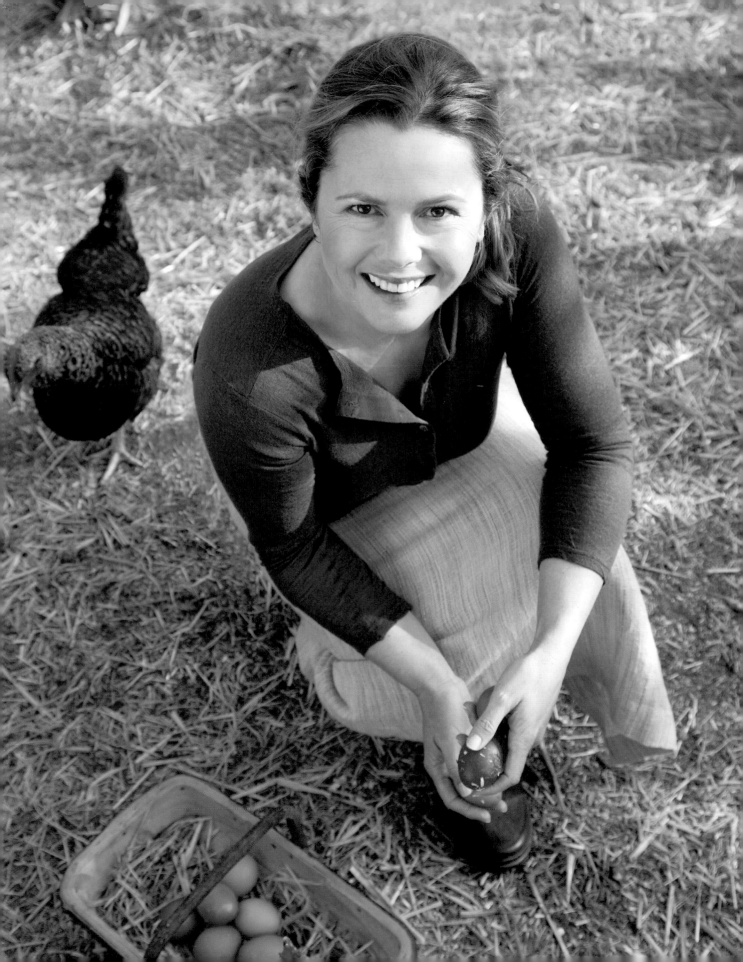

Good eggs and happy hens

So which came first? Either way, it doesn't matter as both chickens and eggs are a healthy, skin-friendly food source.

Eggs are the perfect food, packed with protein, vitamins A, D, E and the stress-busting B-complex vitamins, as well as minerals (iron, phosphorus and skin-building zinc). Organic eggs are especially rich in trace elements, too, such as iodine (required for thyroid hormones), selenium (an important antioxidant) and choline (linked to improved brain function). A medium-sized egg contains around 80 kcals and is relatively low in saturated fat. (And that old myth about eggs raising cholesterol levels is being debunked now, although people with genetically inherited high cholesterol should, of course, check with their doctors.)

Please don't judge an egg by its shell, but by the label on the box. I advocate only free-range (preferably organic), as the production of all other eggs entails an industrial level of production that is incredibly cruel to chickens (as caged or 'barn' hens). I choose organic eggs because the birds are always free-range and fed a varied, nutrient-rich, GM-free diet. Eggs are a by-product of what hens eat, so the better the feed, the healthier the egg. I feed my hens flax seeds (which contain omega-3 and omega-6) and lots of healthy greens – they love brassicas, so I treat them to seasonal sprout tops and the occasional cabbage. They repay me with beautiful, speckled brown shells housing the most

delicious, golden-yolked eggs. If this inspires you to keep your own hens, take a look at a website called www.downthelane.net. Even a small urban space can house an Eglu – a little house plus a small movable run – for a couple of happy hens.

Chicken is also a delicious and healthy, high-protein food, but please choose your chick carefully. Budget, battery chickens are cruelly reared and tasteless (in both senses of the word) to eat. Choose an organic or free-range chicken that comes with giblets inside (which are great to boil into stock for soup). An organic chicken costs more, but goes a long way. My preference is always to buy better-quality meat (and eat it less often), instead of pricier processed meals made with the mechanically recovered grey sludge that masquerades as meat. One good-quality chicken goes a long way – a family meal of roast chicken with all the trimmings at the weekend, leftovers made into a chunky soup or vegetable casserole, a stock boiled from the bones to make a tasty base for broth. And don't forget the iron-rich chicken livers, which I like to save and cook separately, pan-frying in a little olive oil and serving on a slice of spelt or rye toast for a simple – and delicious – lunch or supper.

I choose organic eggs because the birds are always free-range and fed a varied, nutrient-rich, GM-free diet

Milk

I am nearly as passionate about the quality of milk as I am about eggs and chickens. So, here goes!

Milk is a wonderful food and I give my family – including myself – a glass every day to boost skin-building protein and bone-strengthening calcium. Whole milk from organic grass-fed cows contains significant levels of conjugated linolenic acid (CLA), which helps your body metabolise fat and protein, and may have immune-boosting properties. It works by helping to inhibit the enzyme that transports fat from the bloodstream to be stored in fat cells, which is why CLA supplements are touted to help weight loss. CLA may also play a role in reducing cardiovascular disease, by preventing fatty deposits building up in the arteries. If you prefer a lighter taste (as I do), opt for semi-skimmed, as this contains some CLA in the remaining fat. (Skimmed milk contains hardly any.)

Read the label

I always recommend non-homogenised milk (sold by most larger supermarkets) because homogenisation (a mechanical process, in which milk is forced through pipes and fine filters at high speed under pressure) breaks down the fat into tiny particles that are emulsified and suspended evenly throughout the milk, like mist in a fog. These tiny particles allow an enzyme called xanthine oxidase (which would normally be digested into smaller molecules) to pass intact into the bloodstream where it attacks arterial walls and parts of the heart muscle, causing inflammation. Some researchers believe homogenised milk is a significant factor in the rise of heart disease. Shake non-homogenised milk well or skim off the top layer of cream – I serve this separately on fruit crumbles and puddings).

Organic milk gets a gold star, owing to its significantly higher levels of omega-3 Essential Fatty Acids and the skin-supporting antioxidants vitamin E, beta-carotene, lutein and zeaxanthine. The milk is more nutritious because the cows are better fed, spending much of the year grazing in grassy meadows, feasting on a diet high in forage such as fresh clover, wildflowers and hay. You can taste the difference.

Go organic!

Organic dairy cows are never given any animal-derived feeds, thought to be the source of the devastating BSE outbreak, and there has never been a case of BSE found in an organically born and raised dairy cow. It is produced without the routine use of antibiotics and the genetically engineered hormone rBST, banned in Europe, which boosts milk production in cows, but increases cases of mastitis. This condition is not only painful for cows but also more likely to leave traces of pus and antibiotics in the milk, along with a carcinogenic hormone, IGF-1.

The health worries affecting milk extend to all dairy products – good reasons to opt for organic butter, yogurt, cream and cheese, too.

Dairy products may trigger eczema (and acne) in some people, especially small children. A simple exclusion diet – cutting out all dairy products for a week, to see if the skin improves – is a good way to determine this. If you're unable to eat dairy products, other good options include goat, sheep, rice, oat and GM-free soya milks. Encouragingly, babies and children who are intolerant of bovine dairy products usually outgrow this sensitivity. My eldest son could not tolerate cow's milk as a small child and had calcium-enriched rice milk on his cereal for years, but was able to drink cow's milk from the age of about 12.

Interestingly, a large study in The Netherlands of nearly 3,000 atopic patients found that the incidence of eczema in young children was reduced by 36 per cent when they switched to organic dairy products, so switching to organic produce is worth a try, too.

Organic milk gets a gold star,
owing to its significantly higher
levels of omega-3 Essential
Fatty Acids

Beauty breakfasts

Starting with a good breakfast is the best way to boost energy levels for the day ahead and supplies valuable skin-improving nutrients.

Boiled egg

Really, we should all adopt that old ad slogan, 'Go to work on an egg'. Researchers at Louisiana State University found that those who ate two eggs a day for their breakfast lost 65 per cent more weight than the control group (who ate the caloric equivalent in bagels) after six weeks, with no other dietary changes. They concluded the result is down to the fact that eggs give a greater feeling of satiety (as does all protein, compared to carbs or fats), so we tend to eat less during the rest of the day.

Gently place a fresh egg into a small saucepan of rapidly boiling water and cook for between 4–5 minutes (for a medium to large egg) depending on how runny you like yours. Serve with toast soldiers (preferably wholewheat/granary/rye bread) and a shot of vitamin C – in a glass of freshly squeezed orange juice (drunk through a straw to protect tooth enamel), or a bowl of strawberries or slice of cantaloupe melon, to increase your uptake of iron from the egg yolk.

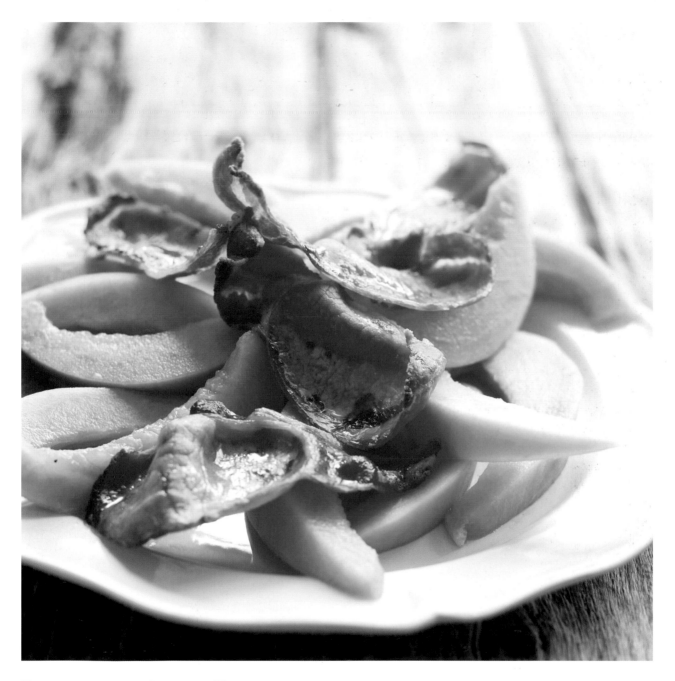

Bacon and melon medley

This is my breakfast/brunch version of the Italian classic of Parma ham and melon. We produce our own bacon from a traditional breed of pig called Oxford Sandy Black, but if I'm buying bacon I always choose organic because of the higher levels of animal welfare, better quality animal feed and lack of artificial growth promoters.

Serves 4

✳ **8 slices unsmoked back bacon**

✳ **1 small cantaloupe melon**

Grill the bacon with the fat on to retain the flavour (trim the fat after cooking it). While this is grilling, de-seed and slice the melon into 16 pieces and arrange on a platter. Place the cooked bacon on top and serve at once. Yum!

Warming winter porridge

This great breakfast dish, which is very quick to make, sets me up for the day when it's cold and dark outside – or any time, actually. Of course, you can just make porridge with rolled oats, but I like the mix of textures here.

Serves 1

* **3 tablespoons whole rolled porridge oats (jumbo-size are good)**
* **2 tablespoons medium oatmeal**
* **150ml water**
* **50ml organic whole milk**

Simply tip all the ingredients into a saucepan and stir over a medium heat for 5–10 minutes. If you like, serve sprinkled with dark brown muscovado sugar.

Fresh fruit salad with yogurt and seeds

Combine half a chopped apple, half a peeled, chopped orange or grapefruit, a few seedless grapes and a handful of seasonal berries. Sprinkle a teaspoonful of sunflower and pumpkin seeds on top and serve with a small (150g) pot of natural yogurt.

Breakfast to go

If I'm in a rush, I spread some protein-rich almond butter between two low-GL oat cakes and take these with me to eat in the car or on the train. High-protein soya yogurts are also 'good to go'.

Apple and yogurt mix

I like this easy-to-make, naturally sweet breakfast any time, but especially during the summer months, when I tend to suffer from hayfever: most cereals aggravate that clogged-up feeling, but this makes me feel clearer-headed and look brighter, too. The nuts and seeds provide skin-friendly Essential Fatty Acids, live yogurt gives the digestive tract a generous helping of beneficial probiotics (to replenish the 'good' bacteria in your gut) and the berries contain important antioxidants called proanthocyanidins, which help prevent the breakdown of collagen and repair any damage.

Serves 1

* **1 apple, preferably organic**
* **4–5 dessertspoons plain live yogurt (full or low fat, or half and half)**
* **1–2 dessertspoons flaked almonds**
* **1 dessertspoon sunflower seeds**
* **1–2 tablespoons berries (optional)**
plus
* **1 tablespoon oats, if you like**

Grate the apple (with the peel on) directly into a bowl.
Spoon in the yogurt.
Stir in flaked almonds and sunflower seeds and the (optional) oats.
Top with any sort of pink, red or blue berry.
Eat it straight away – unless you especially like it soggy, which I don't!

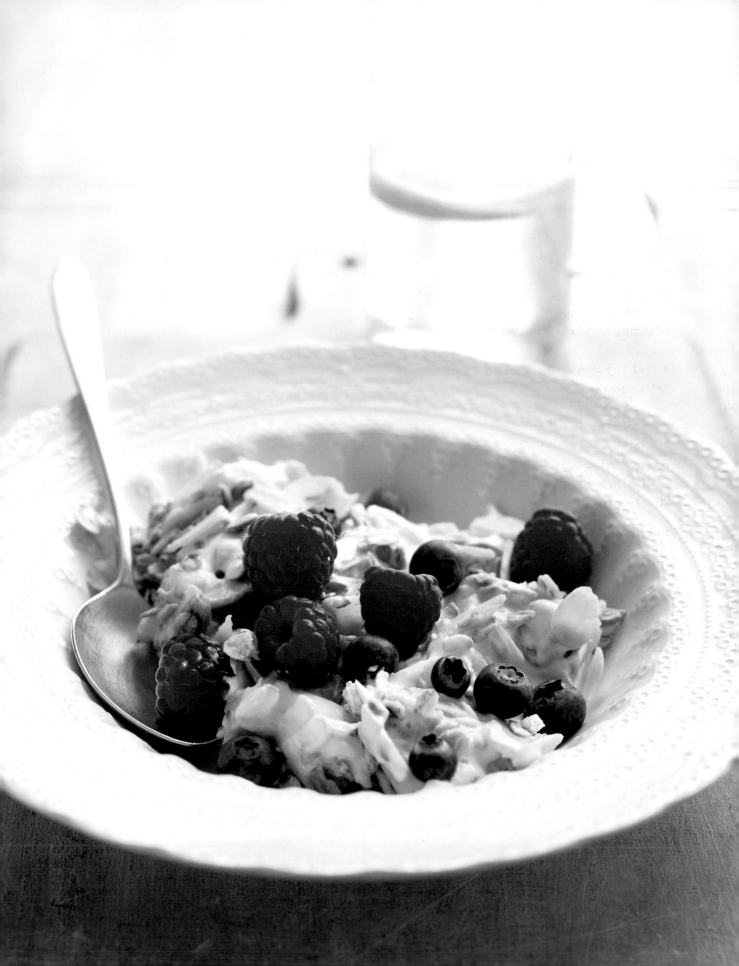

Skin Snacks

Skin loves to be supplied with a steady supply of good nutrients, notably proteins, vitamins, minerals and Essential Fatty Acids from nuts and seeds.

Eating every three hours helps to keep blood sugars stable during a busy day, giving you a bit more vim and vigour and keeping your hormones calm. This trail mix is perfect for a quick energy boost, or for when you need a healthy travel snack. I make a batch every couple of weeks and keep a small pot on my desk and in my travel bag. My children love to raid the tin too.

Trail mix

Simply mix together equal weights of brazil nuts, sunflower seeds, raisins, whole or flaked almonds and pumpkin seeds. (I use 100g of each for a small bag, 200g for a big one.) Add in other goodies as you like, such as chopped dates, dried cherries, cranberries and pomegranate seeds. If all else fails, or I run out, I buy a bag of whole almonds (the kind with their brown skins on) and munch a few of these: almonds are one of the best sources of vegetable protein, high in mono-unsaturated fats and vitamin E, plus the minerals magnesium and potassium.

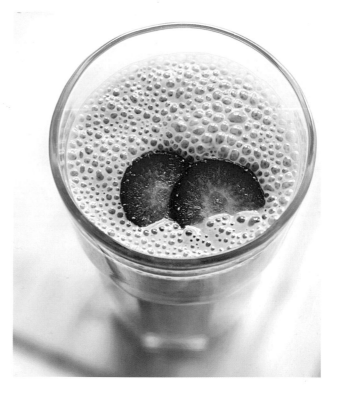

Strawberry smoothie

Smoothies are a delicious way to up your vitamin quota – particularly good for fussy children. In fact, I always have to make double, or my little ones drink it all.

For 1 large glass

* ❋ **12–15 ripe strawberries**
* ❋ **100ml apple juice**
* ❋ **4 tablespoons low-fat, plain live yogurt**
* ❋ **Splash of pomegranate juice (optional)**

Whizz all the ingredients together in a blender, pour into a tall glass, garnish with a few slices of fresh strawberry and enjoy while its cold!

Tip:

Strawberry smoothie makes a great frozen dessert and a healthy low-fat alternative to ice cream.

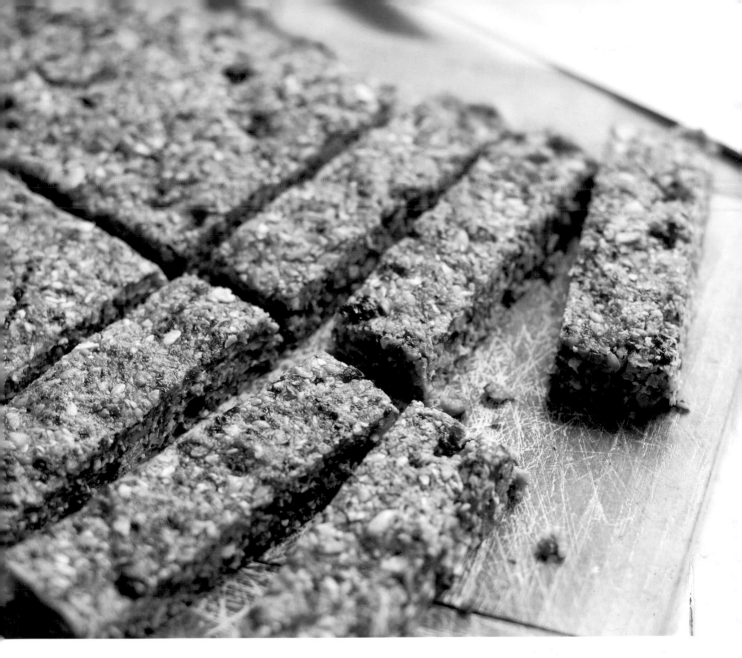

Beauty-boost bars

These terrific omega-rich energy bars are a firm favourite. I make a batch at the weekend and keep them in a sealed box in the fridge for the week ahead – perfect for a post-supper sweet snack, a fast school-run breakfast in the car or for a quick energy boost when blood sugar levels dip, mid-afternoon. I try to keep all these healthy staples in my cupboards, as they are useful for other recipes, too, such as home-made mueslis, biscuits and yogurt toppings.

* **50g each dates, dried apricots, sunflower seeds**
* **100g raisins**
* **100g porridge oats**
* **30g wheatgerm**
* **25g medium oatmeal**
* **20g linseeds**
* **Juice and grated zest of 1 unwaxed lemon**
* **1 tablespoon honey, preferably local**
* **2 tablespoons cold-pressed flax or rapeseed oil, plus a drizzle to grease the tin**

Whizz all the ingredients in a food processor until it forms a firm dough ball. Lightly oil a 20cm loaf tin or one end of a rectangular baking dish. Press the dough into the pan to a thickness of about 2cm. Chill in the fridge for about an hour. Cut into cubes or sticks and enjoy! For a variation, try the juice and zest of an orange instead of lemon.

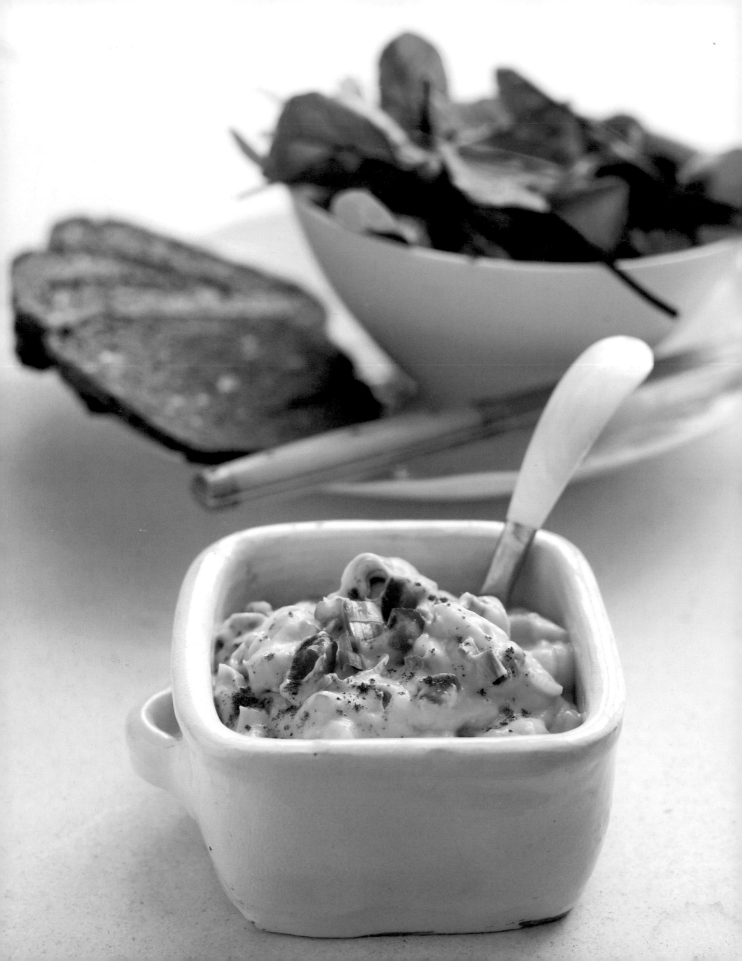

Guacamole

Avocado is naturally rich in vitamin E and skin-saving Essential Fatty Acids and this easy-to-make dip is a healthy snack to enjoy with crudités, oat cakes or rye toast; it also works well with salad, for a summer lunch.

Serves 4

* **1 ripe avocado, flesh scooped into a bowl**
* **30ml/2 tablespoons lemon juice**
* **3 spring onions, finely chopped**
* **2 ripe tomatoes (fresh or tinned), skinned, deseeded and finely chopped**
* **1 clove garlic, peeled and crushed**
* **30ml/2 tablespoons extra virgin olive oil**
* **Tabasco or chilli sauce to taste**
* **Salt and freshly ground black pepper**

Blend the all the ingredients in a food processor until smooth, and decorate with a dusting of paprika and chopped fresh parsley, if you like.

Sesame seed dressing

Tip all these good oils into an empty, clean jam jar, put the lid on tightly and shake well, to mix. Keep in the fridge, where it should last for several weeks, and use liberally on salads, avocados, tomato slices, etc. The high olive-oil content will make the dressing solidify slightly in the fridge, so remove to liquefy at room temperature for a few minutes before using.

Makes 150ml

* **50ml cold-pressed rape seed/flaxseed/hemp oil**
* **50ml extra virgin olive oil**
* **50ml balsamic vinegar**
* **1 teaspoon sesame seeds**
* **1 teaspoon freshly squeezed lemon juice**
* **1 teaspoon runny honey**
* **½ teaspoon salt**
* **½ teaspoon freshly ground black pepper**

Smoked mackerel pâté

Serves 4

This lighter version of a culinary classic is very healthy and extremely skin friendly! Instead of the usual butter or sour cream, I like to use yogurt which is lighter and fresher-tasting.

* **200g smoked mackerel fillets**
* **100ml plain live yogurt**
* **1 tablespoon freshly chopped parsley**
* **1 large garlic clove, crushed and finely chopped**
* **2 teapoons freshly squeezed lemon juice**
* **Salt and plenty of freshly ground black pepper**

Peel away the skin on the mackerel fillets.
In a large bowl, flake the flesh of the fish with a fork and stir in the remaining ingredients, mixing until well combined.
Tip into a bowl and press down with the fork.
Chill for half an hour, then serve with fingers of warm, toasted rye bread, or oatcakes and yogurt.

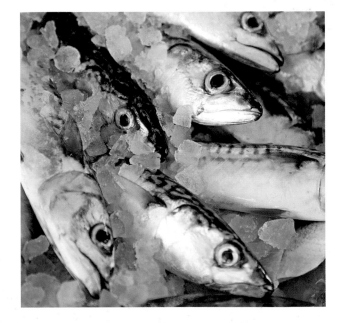

Detox

Even small changes in what we eat and drink can bring about a big difference in the way we look and feel.

The key is to maximise energy-enhancers and minimise energy-sappers. Here are my secrets:

Cut out refined sugar: found in almost everything from breakfast cereals to processed foods and the more obvious cakes, biscuits and sweets. You'll find you have more sustained energy throughout the day instead of bursts of sugar-rush activity followed by a noticeable sugar slump. I switch to porridge in the morning, simply made with water and drizzled with a tiny bit of local honey and a sprinkling of sunflower seeds, for sweetness. Instead of cakes and biscuits, I stock the cupboard with oat cakes or corn thins and spread these with organic peanut or almond butter – a fantastic energy-boosting snack.

Cut down on caffeine: when my caffeine quota creeps up, I redress the balance by swapping rocket-fuel espressos for a gentler cup of decaf or weak tea. However, I don't go cold turkey and give up caffeine altogether, as I find the withdrawal headaches are too debilitating and don't respond to painkillers (not good for the system, in any case). My less draconian detox regime involves cutting down on coffee and strong tea by one cup a day, until I'm down to one small mug at breakfast. Only then, after a week or so of gradual withdrawal, will I give it up altogether.

Substitute fresh herb and spice teas: you can make these great detox boosters for very little at home by infusing boiling water with herbs or spices. Fresh peppermint is an excellent internal cleanser. Simply steep a small bunch of fresh mint leaves in hot water and leave to infuse for a few minutes. It's usually sweet enough to drink without honey and is especially good after meals as a digestion settler and stomach soother – also for bloating, indigestion or general overindulgence.

For a re-energising pep-up, try a few slices of fresh ginger steeped in hot water (sweeten with a little honey, if needed). This is highly anti-bacterial, and is an excellent internal cleanser. I drink lots of it if I'm feeling under the weather, and it really helps. It's also the traditional remedy for nausea or sickness (and even a self-induced hangover).

Take action on alcohol: as with caffeine, I make a tactical retreat over a week or more, gradually making the couple of glasses or so in the evening much smaller, until eventually they're gone altogether, and I haven't felt too deprived. The only thing I'll dramatically increase is drinking water – yes, I know it's an old chestnut, but there's no doubt that drinking much more water (aim for eight large glasses a day) really is a tremendous health, beauty and skin benefit.

Body brushing: the physical process of body brushing is one of the best ways to stimulate a sluggish circulation and help clear built-up toxins from the system. It really gives our internal lymph system a physical boost – which, in turn, increases the amount of cellular debris and waste matter that our lymph system carries out of the body. (See page 13 for more details.)

Sleeeep: if you want to detox effectively, award yourself a peaceful weekend at home, turn the phones and computer off, shut the door and rest as much as you can.

Nutritional Supplements:

These supplements (widely available in health stores) help support your body as you lose fat. Probiotics improve the digestive system, increasing energy and improving metabolism. **Digestive enzymes** help us break down fats, and absorb protein. **Gentle colon cleansing-specific herbs** help detox the body and reduce bloating. Also, **psyllium husks** (swallowed with water) bulk in the colon and help expel waste matter more efficiently.

You can make these great detox boosters
very cheaply at home by infusing boiling
water with herbs or spices

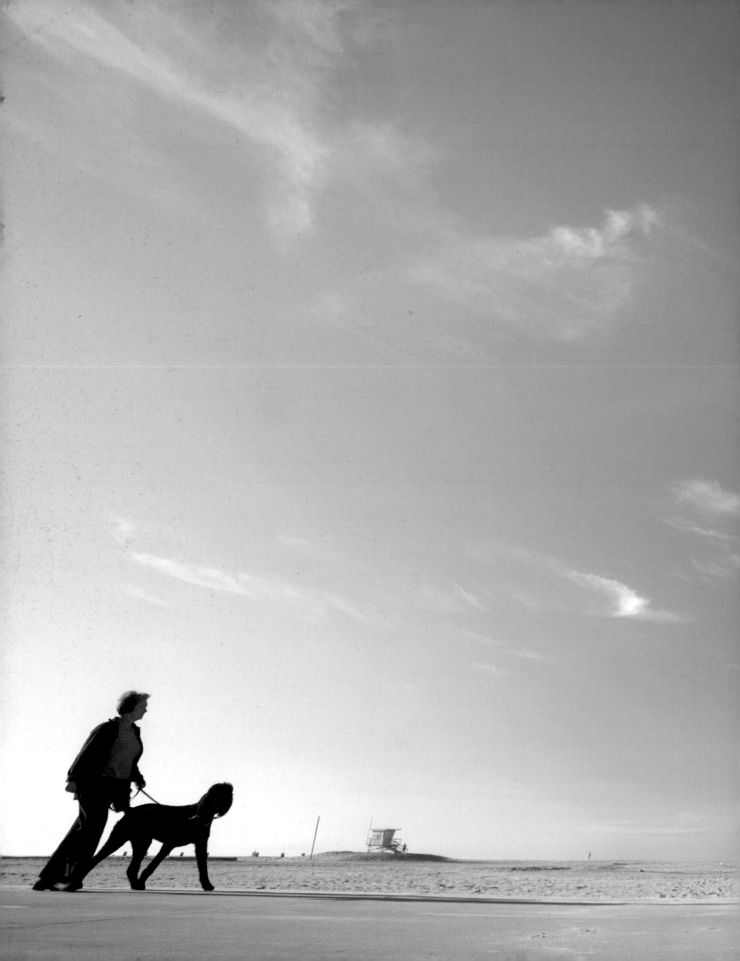

Chapter Eight

EVERYDAY FITNESS

Bodies were designed to move, not sit slumped around. The benefits of daily exercise in terms of general wellbeing, youthful and glowing skin are very visible and real.

Keep it moving

Think how you look – and feel – when you come in from a brisk walk: bright-eyed and sparkling. The simple routines in this chapter are all you need to be like that every day, wherever you are.

Each activity performs a particular task for your body – and many combine more than one. On the following pages, I have used the abbreviations below to indicate what each activity does.
Cardiovascular: works out your heart and lungs; starts to burn fat if you do enough – CV
Weight (or load) bearing: helps your bones – W
Resistance: helps develop muscular strength and prevents you losing muscle mass – R

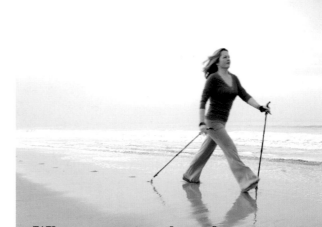

Exercise is every bit as important for your skin as good food and skincare. It increases blood flow, which delivers skin-building nutrients and oxygen supplies to the epidermis. The benefits – pink cheeks, sparkling eyes and radiant glow – are instantly visible. I'm not talking about spending hours in the gym (unless you've the time and inclination), simply doing enough physical activity to leave you slightly out of breath every day. Little and often works best for me. Before I had children, I went to aerobic and Pilates classes: now I fit in 10-minute blocks through the day, starting with my Power Blast.

Getting outside and seeing the changing seasons is a tonic, whether you're in a park in town, or on the seashore. I love Nordic walking either alone or with friends. You use poles to tone and strengthen the upper body and it's fantastic for relieving shoulder tension, plus my skin really glows after a walk-out! (There's more information on the website www.nordicwalking.co.uk)

Aim to do 30–60 minutes at least five days a week. Experts agree you need three different kinds of exercise to keep you fit.

What exercise does for you

❋ Keeps your weight down
❋ Helps keep your body toned and sleek
❋ Keeps you fit – no puffing and panting when you run after your little ones, or a bus
❋ Helps you sleep well
❋ Helps your digestive system work better
❋ Makes your cheeks pink and your eyes sparkle
❋ Helps headaches and fatigue
❋ Puts you in a good mood, lifts anxiety and depression; helps you fight stress
❋ Helps protect you against illness of all kinds, including heart disease, diabetes and breast cancer.
❋ Triggers a woman's adrenal glands to produce a form of oestrogen – nature's own HRT

Experts believe that some of the age-related decline in physical and brain function may be stopped – or even reversed – by regular physical activity.

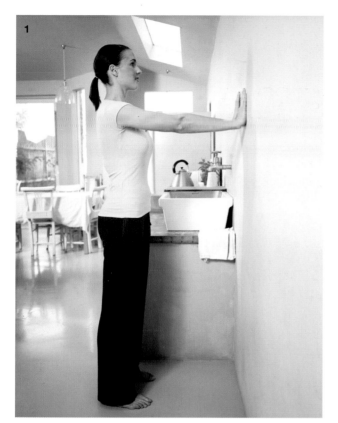

Kettle-boiling stretches

Do these in the morning while the kettle boils... they take two to five minutes, depending on how long you hold for.

(1) Face a wall or door, with your feet about 25cm away from the base. Without leaning on it, stretch your arms up and press your hands into the wall. Working up from your feet, feel your body stretch and align itself: press your thighs back, press your tailbone and shoulder blades towards the wall, squeeze your outer elbows towards each other, and stretch your palms and fingers up. Keep your breathing soft and your jaw relaxed. (30–90 seconds)

(2) Stand facing a chair, hands on hips. Put your right heel on the chair seat. Straighten your left – standing – leg by pressing the thigh back. Let the right leg stretch from hip to heel. Hold for 15 seconds and swap. Do each side twice. Over time, you can work up to putting your heel onto the back of the chair, a table and finally a worktop, but don't rush things – it's never worth it! (1–2 minutes)

(3) Stand by a work top with your hands flat on it, shoulder width apart. Walk your legs slowly back and straighten your arms out until your back is almost parallel with the floor. Your head should be between your arms. You can feel your trunk begin to stretch and your spine realign itself. To help the process, press your thighs back, tuck your tailbone and shoulder blades in, squeeze your elbows towards each other and press your hands down. Keep your breathing soft and your neck and jaw relaxed. Walk towards your hands to come back up. (30–90 seconds)

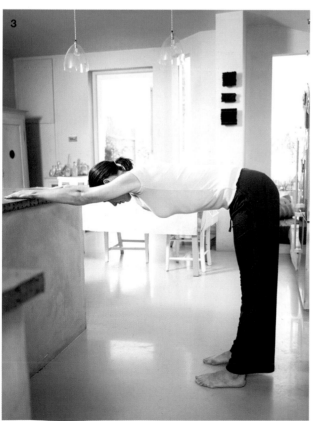

Safety first

To prevent injury, ALWAYS warm up, stretch, exercise, cool/slow down, stretch. Allow 5–10 minutes each to warm up and cool down, depending on how much activity you have done before starting, and the length and intensity you exercise at.

Warming up is simple: walk around the garden for 5 minutes, go up and down stairs or simply get moving around the bedroom.

10-minute Power Blast

I find it best to exercise first thing in the morning, before the day crowds the opportunity. This is my personal plan, which works well wherever I am

I joined Viv Worrall's exercise classes several years ago but, because I'm so busy and often travelling, I see her far less often than I should. To make up for this, Viv gave me this simple set of moves, which I call my '10-minute Power Blast'. I keep the instructions on a card in my suitcase and do them anywhere and everywhere round the globe.

American fitness and weight-loss supremo and bestselling author, Jorge Cruise, claims it takes just 8 minutes of specific exercises in the morning to lose weight, as this is the best time of the day to get your metabolism going. I try never to skimp this Power Blast, as I unfailingly feel better for it: more alert, less stressed and ready to face the day – and with a revved-up metabolism to help keep middle-aged spread at bay.

This is cardiovascular exercise, designed to increase your heart rate as well as tone your shape. If you want to do more, and have time – go for it! But remember that quality is important. Viv keeps reminding me that it's more important to do these exercises precisely for a shorter period than shamble through for half an hour.

For the upper-body exercises you will need two weights. I use 1.5kg dumbbells, but if you don't have a pair, you can use regular-sized tins of baked beans (or anything similar).

As you do each exercise, try to contract the deeper abdominal muscles (your own inner corset) by pulling your navel back to your spine.

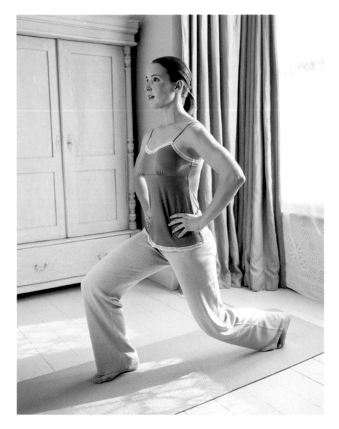

Legs and buttocks
Round-the-clock lunges (CV, W, R)
These are great for strengthening and toning the legs and buttocks, and improving body stability. Going 'round the clock' gives your legs an all-round workout. Start each one with your feet a hip-width apart. Stand straight, looking ahead and breathing evenly. You can take them at a fair lick, but don't skimp on the downward bend, as it's the lunge that works your muscles. These lunges are designed to be done as a sequence. With each, start with 4–6 repetitions on each leg, depending on your strength and fitness; increase by 2 repetitions each, as you feel stronger, building up to 12, if possible – 8, if you get too tired.

Forward lunge (12 o'clock)
What it does: shapes your buttocks and legs
✳ Hands on hips, step forward with your right foot so your

knee is over your foot as you bend at your hips, knees and ankles to lower yourself to the floor.

✳ Only go as low as you can while keeping your posture upright.

✳ Your weight should be evenly balanced between both legs – so keep your upper body centred.

✳ Hold for a second.

✳ Lift your front leg and bring it back to the start position.

✳ Do the same with your left foot.

✳ Watch point: to help your balance, keep your hands on hips throughout; try not to press on your front knee to stand up.

Side lunge (3 o'clock and 9 o'clock)

What it does: shapes and strengthens your buttocks, legs, hips and calves, and gives a great stretch for inner thighs

✳ With both feet facing forward, step your right leg right out to the side.

✳ Turn your right foot at a right angle, to avoid straining your lower back.

✳ Bend your right knee, keeping it over your right foot.

✳ Hold for a second before lifting your leg and bringing it back to the start position.

✳ Do the same with your other leg.

Reverse lunge (6 o'clock)

What it does: tones and tightens buttocks and legs

✳ Step back with your right leg and bend at the hips, knees and ankles to lower yourself to the floor.

✳ Only go as low as you can while keeping your posture upright.

✳ Keep your left (front) knee over your left mid-foot.

✳ Your weight should be evenly balanced between both legs – so keep your upper body centred.

✳ Hold for a second before lifting your back leg and bringing it back to the start position.

✳ Do the same with your left leg.

Upper arms
Bicep curls (R)

What it does: shapes and strengthens upper arms especially biceps (front of arm)

✳ Stand with feet hip-width apart.

✳ With arms down by your sides, grasp a dumbbell – or tin – in each hand, palms upward.

✳ Bend your elbows (leave your upper arms by your sides) and lift the weights up to your shoulders; hold for a second before slowly lowering back to start.

✳ Aim for 8–10 repetitions.

✳ Watch point: keep your upper body still and your tummy held in, and don't stop breathing!

✳ Slow the moves right down and you will really feel the muscle fibres working.

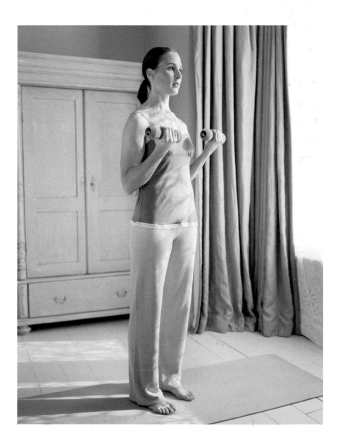

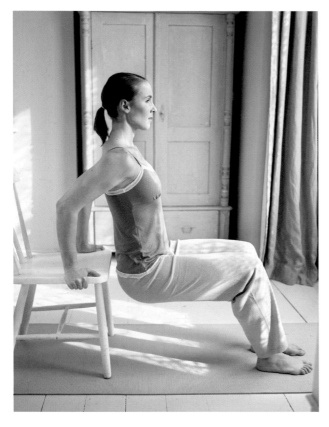

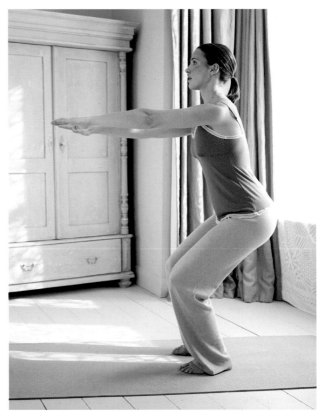

Tricep dips (W, R)

What it does: strengthens and tones the shoulders and back of upper arms (triceps). But you need to be reasonably fit to do this

✳ Sit on the edge of a stout chair, hands holding the sides.

✳ Stretch your legs straight out in front, heels resting on the floor.

✳ Taking your weight on your arms, lift your bottom up and slightly forward from the chair.

✳ Bending arms and knees, lower yourself towards the floor, as far as you can go, feeling safe and secure.

✳ Lift yourself up by straightening your arms and legs.

✳ Start with 2–6 repetitions and build up to 8–12.

✳ **Watch point:** it's really important the chair is solid enough not to move at all. (Try positioning it firmly against the wall.)

Squats (C, W, R)

What it does: develops strength in the lower body, helps improve balance and stability; also helps shape and define buttocks

✳ Stand with your feet hip-width apart, feet pointing forwards.

✳ With your back straight, bend your knees – pushing your hips back and down, as if to sit down.

✳ Keep your weight even in the middle of your feet, and only go as low as you feel in control.

✳ To help you balance, reach your arms straight out in front, and focus on a distant point.

✳ Hold for a second before coming up slowly and with control: imagine you are pushing your feet into the floor.

✳ Squeeze your buttocks on the way back up.

✳ Start with 4–6 repetitions and build up to 8–12.

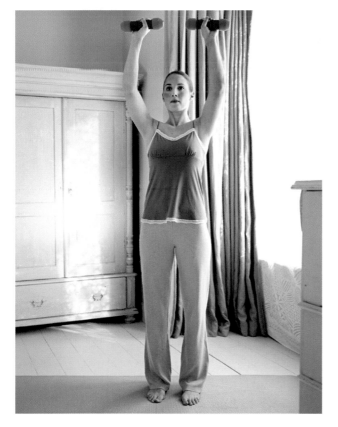

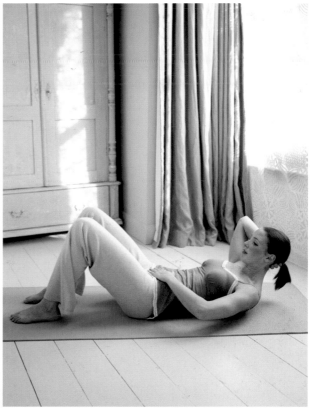

Overhead press (R)

What it does: shapes and sculpts your shoulders

✳ Stand with your feet hip-width apart, knees slightly bent.

✳ Hold a weight at shoulder height in each hand, with your palms facing forward and down, upper arms by your side and elbows bent.

✳ Keep your navel pulled back towards your spine.

✳ Push the weights up above your head towards the ceiling. (But don't bend your neck backwards.)

✳ Bring them back to start and repeat.

✳ Aim for 8–10 repetitions.

✳ **Watch point:** don't let your shoulders rise to your ears as you lift the weights.

Pilates curl-ups (R)

What it does: strengthens the abdominal muscles and helps flatten your stomach

✳ Lie on your back on the floor, feet hip-width apart.

✳ Cup the back of your head with your right hand.

✳ Rest your left hand, palm down, on your lower abdominal muscles.

✳ As you do this exercise, imagine you are pulling your navel back from your hand towards your spine.

✳ Lift your head, then your shoulders off the floor and curl up towards your navel.

✳ Try not to tilt your pelvis and keep your abdominals flat.

✳ If you are comfortable with that, lift your upper body higher by bringing your breastbone towards your navel too.

✳ Hold for a second, then uncurl very slowly.

✳ Start with 4 repetitions (2 with each hand), slowly building up to 12 repetitions total.

✳ **Watch point:** keep your neck and shoulders soft, and don't pull your chin into your chest.

Slow-down stretches

The secret of a stress-free face is to release as much tension as possible before it builds up in the rest of your body.

Do these simple exercises any time you need to slow down and unkink your body. You could have a little session when you've finished your Power Blast, or when you feel in need of physical soothing and smoothing. (If you're away from home you might want to omit the ones where you lie on the floor.) I like to do them in the evening, before I go to bed, especially if I am travelling and really need to wind down.

Shoulder rolls – to release tension from your upper body: Stand comfortably, or do them sitting at your desk or in a car, on a train or plane.

Roll your shoulders back and round – and round, and round… Say, 6 times. Then repeat, rolling forwards.

Upper-body stretch – to lengthen your spine and free the discs and muscles:

Again, you can do this standing or sitting.

✳ Lace your fingers together in front of you, palms facing towards you.

✳ Raise your arms to the ceiling, turning your palms upward as you go.

Side bend – extends each side of your body:

✳ Standing or sitting, with your feet a hip-width apart and knees soft, reach your arms to the ceiling, palms forward. Then bend like a windmill to your right, feeling the stretch down the left side of your body. Repeat on the left side.

Roll down (1) – this is one of my favourite Pilates-inspired stretches to mobilise the spine and release tension:

✳ Stand with your feet a hip-width apart, knees soft.

✳ Gently drop your chin towards your chest, then slowly roll forward through every part of your spine, going from top to bottom. Let your knees bend slightly as you go. Remember to draw your navel in towards your spine.

✳ Let your head, arms and upper body hang like a rag doll near your slightly bent knees.

✳ Bring your head towards your knees: roll down as far as you comfortably can. You are aiming to let your body rest

on your thighs, with the backs of your hands on the floor. You may feel a stretch in the back of your legs.

✳ When you can go no further, breathe in, and on the out breath, very gently start to roll yourself up – 'restacking' your spine from the base up.

Thread the needle (2) – this is the best exercise I've found to release tension in my upper back

✳ Kneeling on all fours, lift your right hand, palm upward, and reach it under your left armpit, pointing out to the side – as it were, at 9 o'clock

✳ Let your right shoulder and face dip towards the floor; allow your left elbow to bend as you do this, and the shoulder to relax.

✳ Rest for 10–12 seconds with your right shoulder and the right side of your face on the floor. If you're in a dusty place, you might want to put a towel down first!

Or try this simple shoulder stretch instead, which you can do sitting at your desk or on a train or plane. Take your right arm across your body, under your left armpit and reach for your left shoulder blade; put your left arm on top and reach for the right side – as if you are giving yourself a big hug. Hold for a moment, breathing deeply, then swap arms and repeat.

Spinal twist (3) – this is my all-time favourite tension buster – especially for releasing your lower back, if you've been sitting for hours.

✳ Lie flat on your back, knees bent and feet together.

✳ Stretch your arms out to the side from your shoulders, so your body makes the shape of a cross.

✳ Gently drop your knees to your left side as far as you comfortably can, turning your head to look over your right shoulder.

✳ Stay in this position for 2–3 slow breaths, or as long as you like to.

✳ Repeat on the other side.

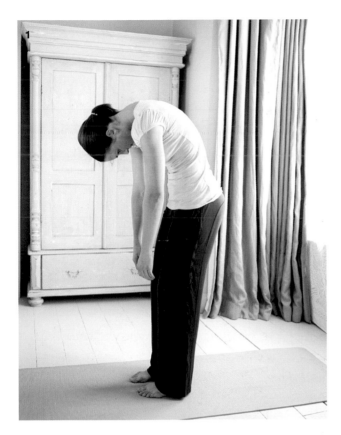

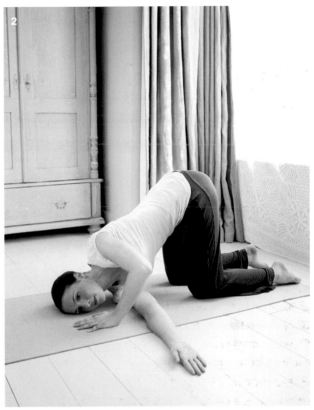

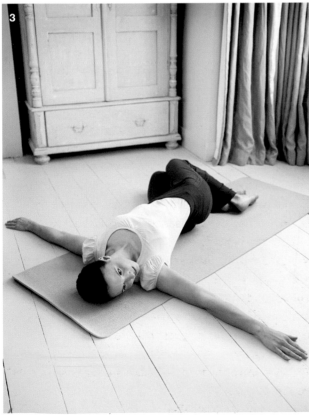

Top-to-toe stretch:

✳ Lie on your back, with your arms behind your head, stretched out straight on the floor.

✳ Point your fingertips away from your head, and your toes in the opposite direction.

✳ Breathe rhythmically and feel your spine open and lengthen.

✳ **Now:** make your hands into fists and simultaneously flex your feet, bringing the toes towards you and pushing the heels away.

✳ Feel the stretch down the back of your legs.

✳ Repeat the whole sequence two to three times.

✳ Finish by letting your whole body relax and go floppy, sinking into the floor. Let your feet fall apart in a V-shape and bring your hands near your sides.

✳ Come up slowly to a sitting position. Take a deep breath in, then slowly breathe out. Repeat for 3 breaths, focusing on your breathing, and feeling any residual tension ebb away.

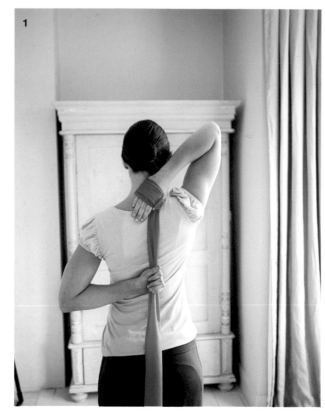

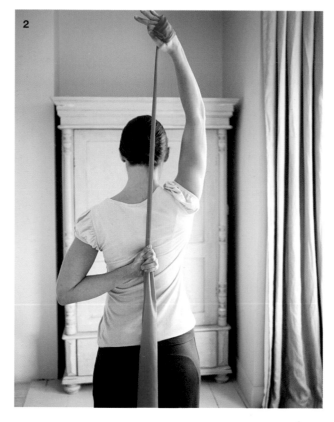

Band aid

You don't need big pieces of high-tech equipment for a gym-type workout: these simple, inexpensive options work a treat.

Resistance exercise, which uses your own body weight, and/or additional weights, or aids such as elastic or a resistance band, is essential for strengthening bones and muscles; it also helps keep you lean and fit by metabolising your body's sugar stores, ready to burn off fat (which, like most people, I have to keep an eye on). I find easily portable, low-tech equipment in the shape of resistance bands (just like giant elastic bands) and soft mini-balls very helpful, especially when I am away from home.

Exercising with a resistance band (R)

These bands come in varying levels of intensity, designated by different colours. I use a medium-resistance band, while my husband and teenage son use tougher ones with greater resistance. Always ensure you have a good hold of

the band before starting each exercise – wrap the ends round your fingers, if necessary. Aim to do each exercise eight to ten times. Warning: to avoid any possibility of injury, do warm up first by doing the same exercises without the band.

Lateral pull-down: to shape and tone your back, and free your shoulders:

✳ Lightly wrap the band ends round each hand, and reach your arms up over your head. Holding the band about a shoulder-width apart, adjust it until there is a slight tension in the elastic.

✳ Then pull your hands away from each other, reaching your arms out and down to shoulder height, until the band is in front of your face.

✳ Slowly move your hands back to the start position.

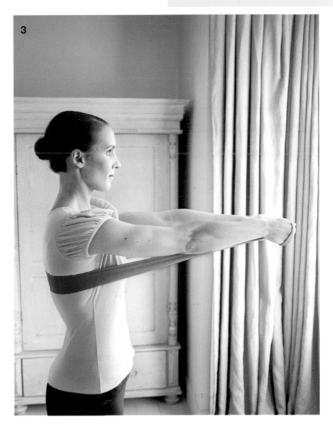

Tricep press (1-2): to tone the backs of your arms:

* Wrap the band firmly round your right hand, and reach your right arm straight up to the ceiling.
* Bend the right elbow and bring your right hand towards the centre of your back between your shoulder blades, letting the loose end of the band fall down your back.
* Reach behind with your left arm. Bend the elbow and reach your left hand as far up the band as you can, towards your right hand.
* Grasp the band and pull: you should feel a slight tension.
* Holding your left hand still, to anchor the band, slowly straighten your right arm and reach your hand upwards towards the ceiling.
* Hold for a second before slowly bending your right arm, and bringing it your hand between the shoulder blades.
* Do 4–6 repetitions with your right arm, building up to 8–12 repetitions. Then swap arms.

Chest press (3): to firm chest area:

* Hold the band loosely in both hands behind your back, about chest height, with the ends hanging down.
* Bend your elbows and, with your hands at shoulder height, wrap the bands securely round each hand. You should feel a slight tension in the band.
* Push your hands forward so your arms are straight out in front of your shoulders.
* Hold for a second, then slowly bend your elbows and bring hands back to your shoulders. Repeat 8–12 times.

Leg press (4): to tone your buttocks and top of legs:

* Lie flat on the floor with knees bent.
* Lift your right foot, keeping the leg bent, and place the middle of the band round the sole.
* Wrap the ends of the band round each hand until you feel a slight tension.
* With your upper arms lying on the floor, bend your elbows until your lower arm and hand are vertical, pointing to the ceiling.
* Push your right leg away until its straight along the floor.
* Slowly bend your knees and release the band.
* Repeat 8–12 times on your right leg. Repeat with left leg.

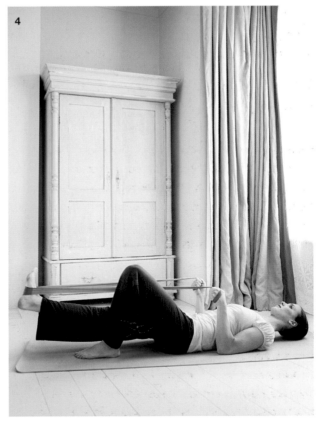

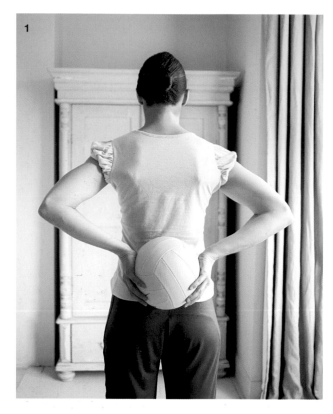

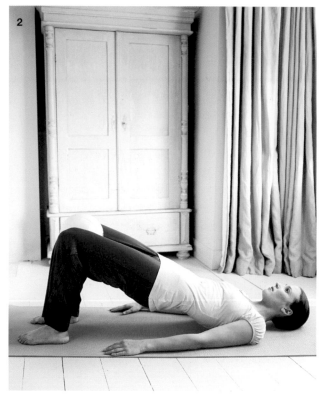

Play ball

I've recently discovered soft mini-balls – about the size of a football – which are really useful to exercise with, both at home and away as they deflate and flat-pack. I use them mainly for stretches, and also as a good head and neck support when I'm exercising lying down. You'll find them in sports shops, or online: for more information, try www.ballsnbands.com; or visit BUPA's online shop and click on Therapy Ball: www.shop.bupa.co.uk/exercise_balls

Chest squeeze (1) – to strengthen arms and back, and stretch chest area (R):
✳ Hold the ball between your palms behind your lower back. Then squeeze the ball by pressing palms towards each other. Hold for one to two seconds. To increase the intensity of the stretch, lift your hands a little way from your body: only go as far as is comfortable.

Buttock lift with inner-thigh squeeze (2) – to tone bottom and inner thighs (R):

✳ Lie on your back, legs together, feet flat on the floor, knees bent. Hold the ball between your knees. Lift your bottom off the floor and hold for one to two seconds. To increase the intensity, squeeze inner thighs together and tighten your bottom muscles.

Half-roll back – to strengthen tummy muscles (R):
✳ Sit on the floor with your knees bent and feet flat on the floor.
✳ Put the ball on the floor just behind your lower back.
✳ Lightly holding the sides of your thighs for support, tilt your pelvis and press your lower back into the ball.
✳ Imagine creating a 'C-shape' with your spine.
✳ Pull your navel towards your spine as you curl into the ball (and also as you come back to the start position).
✳ Hold the pose for one to two seconds.
✳ Come back to the start position, remembering to press your navel towards your spine.
✳ Repeat 4–8 times.

Water workout

(C, R, partial W, if in shallow water)

I love exercising in water because it feels more like a holiday break!

I am not a great swimmer so, instead of doing lengths, I use these simple moves. I appreciate being able to work out while the rest of the family are splashing about nearby.

Aqua aerobics is a thorough workout for the whole of your body, at the same time as being gentle on your joints. Because water is buoyant and supports you, it's suitable for people of all ages and varying abilities. Join a class locally, if you can, or try these simple exercises.

To avoid picking up infections in a swimming pool, wear neoprene beach shoes, or cotton ankle socks. Chlorine is a disinfectant and harsh on the hair and skin, so find a saline or ozone-purified pool, if possible.

Aqua exercises

Do these simple moves in shallow water which comes up to between your navel and nipple line. While you are doing them, remember to keep your shoulders relaxed and let your shoulder blades drop down, while your chest floats upwards. Don't arch your back, though: you may need to lean slightly forwards as you move. Keep pressing your heels to the pool bottom and remember to pull your tummy button back to your spine to help strengthen your abdominal muscles.

Make the exercise more challenging by using buoyant equipment such as handbuoys (buoyant dumb-bells) or noodles (woggles – lengths of soft flexible cylindrical foam, about 165cm long x 7cm diameter). Wearing neoprene shoes or socks also helps to increase the intensity by providing traction as you push off the pool bottom. These are available online from www.hydro-actif.co.uk

Do 8–10 seconds and gradually build up to half a minute. All the moves should increase your heart rate.

Jogging: to strengthen and tone legs:
* Jog as you would on land, lifting your knees as high as you can to your hips, and air-punching the arm opposite to the leg you're lifting.
* You can jog on the spot, or – for more intensity – travel

Handy tips:

You can increase or decrease the intensity of the action by altering your hand position. The harder you push and pull against the water, the harder your workout and the more it will tone your body.
* **Cupping/palming:** open and slightly cup your hand (as you do in most swimming strokes), scooping the water with your palm to increase the intensity.
* **Punching:** make a fist to increase resistance a little, and to add power to your arm movements.
* **Slicing:** slice your hand sideways through the water for less resistance.

forward, pushing your body through the water.
Watch point: keep your body upright and pull your navel back to your spine

Jumping Jacks: to strengthen and tone inner and outer thighs, and shape back and arms:
* Start with your legs together and arms at your sides.
* Jump your legs wide out to each side, and lift your arms as high as you can, but still under water.
* Jump legs back to start position, at the same time pulling your arms back to your sides.

Cross-country ski: to tone legs, arms and torso:
* Step your right leg forward in stride position.
* Reach forward with your left arm and stretch your right arm behind you. Jump your left leg forward, right arm forward and left arm back. Jump back to change position.
* You can do this on the spot or moving forward, if you feel like putting in more effort.

Ski jump: to tone abdominal muscles, hips and arms:
* Start with your feet together.
* Bend your knees and lift feet off the bottom.
* Land feet to the right of centre.
* Lift your feet again and land to the left of centre.
* As you jump to one side, stretch your arms out and across your body, pushing the palms through the water towards the opposite side.

Chapter Nine

RELAX, UNWIND, SLEEP...

Look at your face when you're not worried
and you've had a good night's sleep. Compare
it with a day when you've been stressed and
under pressure, or the morning after a bad
night's sleep. No contest is there? Here
are the tried and tested strategies
I have discovered over the years.

Calm down and make life easier for yourself

Stop … Breathe… Be calm

If you're feeling fussed, stressed, anxious – do something very simple now. Stop. That's it. Just S-T-O-P. The world can manage without you for 5 minutes. And you will manage much better if you take a break.

Sit down, if possible, or stand evenly, with your weight on the middle of your feet. Start breathing – slowly, gently, rhythmically. Inhale through your nose to a count of four, hold it for one or two (more, if you can – the optimum is seven), then exhale through your mouth to a count of six to eight – the slower, the better. Let your shoulder blades sink downwards, and your crown and chest float upwards. Soften your whole body from your jawline to your toes.

Clear your mind. As you get more practised with this 'retention-breathing' technique, close your eyes and imagine yourself in a scene you like and find peaceful. In my mind's eye, I like to 'go' to a sandy beach, watching the waves ebbing and flowing. I can feel the sun warm on my skin, a breeze playing across my frowny forehead – and the tension seeping out of my face and body.

Breathe in time with the waves. Inhale as you watch them creeping up the beach. Hold your breath just as the waves hover before receding (without letting your shoulders rise or your muscles tense). Then exhale as the waves turn and flow back. Repeat 5 or 6 times, twice a day. Do this whenever you are stressed; it's also very effective if you can't sleep, or wake in the small hours.

When you have finished your breathing sequence, go back to your list of priorities – and if you haven't made one, get one done! – and work through them methodically. If you feel yourself getting anxious again, take five: take a breath, go for a little walk. You will feel better and do everything more easily.

Secret

This really recharges your batteries: Stuff two tennis balls into a cotton sock and knot tightly at the top. Lie flat on the floor with the sock under the base of your skull, where the head joins the neck. Relax for no more than 5 minutes. This helps 'switch off' the inner pulse of the cranium and rebalance it, according to cranial osteopath Tamara de Bardi. I find it works.

My five-minute fingertip facelift

If I am tired and headachey at the end of the day, I do this 5-minute routine, which is fantastic for de-stressing the head and reviving your complexion. You can use any facial oil or moisturiser, as the most important part is the lymphatic drainage movements. Lymph fluid moves all over the body, collecting toxins and unwanted cell debris and returning them to the blood circulation to be dealt with. If the process slows up – which it does naturally, overnight, or through exposure to pollutants, lack of exercise or a poor diet – it causes puffiness. These small but precise moves help speed the flow of lymph through your face, immediately helping to reduce eye bags, boost blood circulation and encourage skin cell renewal.

First, thoroughly cleanse and tone your skin, before finding somewhere comfortable and peaceful to sit, perhaps in front of a dressing table or bathroom mirror.

Step 1:

Apply a generous amount of facial oil or moisturiser to your palm and gently warm between both hands. Take a momont to stop, breatho dooply and inhalo the aroma. Let your shoulders fall downwards and clear your mind. Scoop the oil or cream with your fingertips and apply first to the décolleté (above your bosom). Work up the neck and face with the fingertips of both hands, using upward and outward movements. Press quite firmly, but comfortably. Notice any tense or sore spots, such as around the jaw and temples, and apply a little more pressure: also, take a few deep breaths to help the knots release.

Step 2:

With the tips of your middle and ring fingers, start from the bridge of the nose and lightly stroke around the eyes, using sweeping movements upwards and around the sockets, along the rim of the orbital bones. Repeat several times.

Step 3:

Next, with your ring fingers, gently press from the inner corners of the eyes, using fingertip tapping movements to work down and out across the curve of the cheekbones, up past your temples to the outer edge of your eyebrows. Repeat 3–4 times – more, if you have more time.

Step 4:

Using the tips of your thumbs and forefingers, gently pinch along each eyebrow, starting at the bridge of the nose and working outwards. Repeat at least twice. I learnt to do this particular move before TV shows and it really helps to temporarily lift the brows and give the face a mini 'lift'.

Step 5:

Finish by gently sweeping your fingertips up over the upper chest, neck, jaw and cheeks. When working on the chest and neck, it's easiest to alternate one hand after the other, moving from side to side. Then put both sets of fingertips on your chin and sweep fingertips and palms up over your jaw and cheekbones.

Step 6:

Take a few moments to rotate your shoulders; also let your head droop from side to side and massage the upper neck area to relieve stiffness and tension. Finish by consciously relaxing your face – letting go of every tense, tired muscle – so any lines and furrows soften.

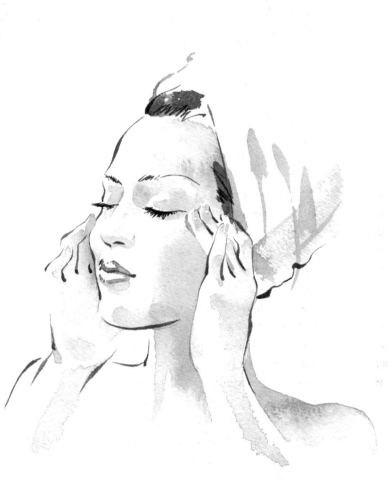

Tip

I am hooked on specially shaped neck cushions, filled with wheat and scented with soothing lavender, which you warm in a microwave or Aga. They're so comforting – excellent for any sort of pain in the neck.

My tried and tested stressbusters

Get outside: when I'm at home on our farm, I head outside first thing in the morning for a brisk walk – even in the cold and grey, it's amazing how energising and exhilarating this is. Most outdoor physical activities are effective stress busters: running, kicking a football, playing with a dog, cycling, horse riding, canoeing, sailing – all have that feeling of wind-in-the-hair release and freedom. If you can't get outside, at least get to a window and pause for a moment to take in the view. I try to see the horizon every day, even if I'm working in a city.

Hugs! Aim for three hugs a day. I'm very lucky that I almost always have family around to clasp, but if you are on your own, do see if you can find friends or pets to cuddle. And when you do, just notice the effects: you stop holding your breath, your shoulders go down, and you start smiling!

Watch comedies: DVDs of Fawlty Towers, Absolutely Fabulous and Frasier never fail to cheer me up on even the stressiest day. Even reading a funny book, or sharing a joke, does the trick: smiling and laughing release feel-good hormones called endorphins in the brain, which scud round the body, literally enhancing our wellbeing.

Surround yourself with positivity, which includes such simple things as looking at pictures of people and pets you love. Because we subliminally absorb what we are surrounded by, even apparently small positives can have a significant impact.

Make a joyful, uplifting playlist on your mp3 player, or tape/CD for the car. Have a good singalong or dance round the kitchen. My feelgood choices include *Kissing Your Cares Goodbye* by The Newsboys, *Shine a Light* by The Mavericks and Abba's *Dancing Queen*.

Take a shower and visualise all the toxic garbage in your mind and body running off you and down the drain. For a really thorough de-stress and detox, I always wash my hair, too. Give your head a firm scalp massage when you apply the shampoo and conditioner, rotating your fingertips from nape to forehead. Finish with a cold rinse – all over! Your reward will be shiny hair and a clear, tension-free head.

Find your faith: several studies have shown that those who follow a spiritual path, usually involving prayer and/or meditation, live longer, healthier and happier lives. I have found my Christian faith brings lasting contentment and a genuine sense of peace, and makes me better able to deal with struggles in life, from fundamental big issues to daily annoying gripes. Many people also find fulfilment in volunteering, joining a choir or music group and fundraising or mission work to help others.

Complementary de-stressers that work for me

Massage: Almost any sort of massage can be relaxing and beneficial. Aromatherapy is wonderful if you, like me, love the experience of being massaged with fragrant essential oils. Manual lymphatic drainage massage (MLD) is great for cellulite. I am also very impressed by a bodywork technique called myofascial release, a 'tender' mixture of stretches and massage techniques. It is especially good for releasing areas of tension held in the body such as neck, shoulders and spine. (All you need is a simple firm foam roller; I use a 15cm x 90cm size from www.physiosupplies.com)

Osteopathy and cranial osteopathy: I'm a fan of osteopathy in general and cranial osteopathy in particular. Where osteopathy focuses on diagnosing and correcting the alignment of the skeleton, cranial (and cranio-sacral, which is slightly different) osteopathy is described as a subtle treatment that releases stresses and tensions throughout the body, including the head. It works on the body's subtle rhythms to re-balance and refresh.

Reflexology: I find this very effective diagnostically for picking up minor (and sometimes not so small) ailments and problems, and to help calm, relax and re-energise – a rare combination. It involves applying pressure to the feet, and sometimes hands, and is based on a system of zones and reflex areas that are said to reflect an image of the body on the feet and hands. By pressing specific areas, it is said to have an effect on the organ concerned.

Secret

Don't look down! Doctors agree that looking up and forward can help ward off depression. Iyengar yoga teacher Hannah Lovegrove says you can't be in a negative mood if you stretch your arms above your head – try it: I think she has something there.

A sweet night's sleep

Sleeping well can not only make us look ten years younger, we can cope with everything better the following day.

As I wrote at the beginning of this book, beauty sleep is just that – beautifying – and an uninterrupted seven hours has been shown to be the optimum. But your bedroom is more than just a place to sleep in. My bedroom is my personal space – well, maybe my husband's too, but I chose the décor. It is painted in my favourite shade of calming eau-de-nil green and has beautiful matching linen curtains. In the corner, there is a small sofa piled with comfy cushions and an old favourite cashmere blanket, and I retreat here for a power nap when pressures pile up. I also have a 'Please do not disturb' sign, which my children made me for the door – very useful.

Your bedroom is your sanctuary, so never take a laptop or other computer into it! (No, not even your Blackberry.)

Not only does this cyber-invasion turn your retreat into an office, it creates electromagnetic radiation, which can disturb sleep patterns. Televisions do the same so, if you must have them, always unplug at the mains socket before sleep – but preferably don't have them at all. I find a radio less intrusive and more soothing.

Don't drink caffeinated drinks (tea, coffee, cocoa, cola, etc) or eat anything very sugary after teatime.

Have a glass or two of good wine: I don't advocate drinking strong spirits but a sociable glass of wine or two with family and friends is a good way to unwind. However, as alcoholic drinks are (bizarrely) sold without any ingredient labelling, I always buy organically produced wines, as these are produced to tight regulations with

Tip

I'm a great list maker, with a 'To Do' list always on the go. When you're very busy, it really focuses your mind on priorities and helps you feel in control – and can help you sleep. Ticking things off your 'To Do' list is so very satisfying.

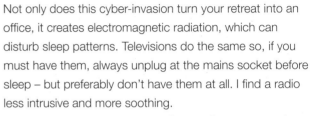

respect to their artificial additive content. Unfortunately, until the drinks industry is properly regulated in favour of the consumer, we simply have no idea what we're imbibing. I regard this as far more worrying than the ingredients we put onto the surface of our skin.

Tip a cupful of old-fashioned (and cheap!) Epsom salts – magnesium sulphate – into the bath. Magnesium is known as 'nature's tranquilliser' – it's also needed for over 300 biochemical reactions in the body – but most of us don't get enough through our diet. According to medical researcher and mother of four Dr Paula Baillie-Hamilton, 'the salts are absorbed through the skin and are brilliant for stress and for aches and pains.' She adds that they're great for children, too: 'Topping up their levels of these compounds really helps them with schoolwork – particularly one child who has learning difficulties.'

Lavender has a truly sedating aroma and has been shown in studies to help relax and quieten brain activity. I keep a small bottle of the essential oil beside my bed and sprinkle a few drops onto a tissue to tuck under my pillow. You can also try adding a few drops to a warm (not hot) bath: breathe in deeply as you step in.

Before you go to sleep, write down in a special notebook all the nice things that have happened during the day (or week, if it's been a bad few days). If you are very busy, also make an action plan for the next day, so you don't wake up panicking at 4am.

Snuggle up to someone you love: giving and receiving love must be the biggest de-stresser ever!

Get a good mattress: we spend so much time on our beds that it really is worth investing in one.Buy the best mattress you can afford and remember to replace it every ten years or so. (If that feels spendthrift, remember you will spend a third of your life on it.) I find the moulded foam-style pillows, such as Tempur, give good neck support. Treat yourself to a special set of fine cotton sheets (the thread count to aim for is 400) and a natural sheepskin mattress topper which, curiously, will keep you cool in summer and warm in winter, as well as cushioning any achey joints or back.

Ideally, you should take five minutes or so to fall asleep from the time you turn out the light – if you fall asleep the instant your head hits the pillow, you are probably overtired and overdoing things. I have found several helpful products for insomnia, include Nytol herbal supplements (with hops, passiflora and wild lettuce) and herbal teas, particularly chamomile, valerian and passiflora.

If you are a light sleeper woken by the slightest noise, try earplugs. The most comfortable and sound proofing are the soft, flexible, silicone kind sold for swimmers. They are especially useful to get a better rest on long-haul night flights or when away from home.

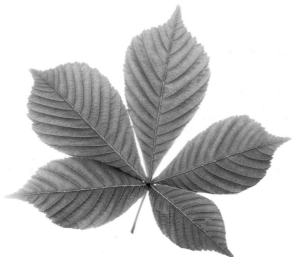

A final word

Beauty is much more than skin deep, but I have always believed that healthy, radiant skin is the icing on the cake. More importantly, whatever our age or stage in life, great looking skin gives our self-esteem a boost, feels more comfortable to live in and causes fewer health problems as we grow older. I hope this book goes some way to help you achieve naturally beautiful skin – easily and without huge expense (financial or time). After all, there are far more important things in life than stressing about how our skin looks. In my own experience, after many years of research and conversations with literally thousands of women around the world, all any of us want is to be free from worrying about the state of our skin. Having good skin is very liberating and the aim of this book is for all skins – regardless of age, type or colour – to look and feel better.

Liz Earle

Liz Earle

2009

Shopping directory

A

* Anti-Allergy Bedcovers, Alprotec Allergy Technologies Ltd,
tel: +44 (0) 161 998 1999,
www.allergy.uk.com
* Aqua aerobic equipment,
tel: +44 (0) 1983 840 555,
www.hydro-actif.com
* Arezoo Kaviani,
tel: +44 (0) 20 7584 6868,
www.arezoo.co.uk

B

* Barbara Daly make up, available at Tesco Customer Service, tel: +44 0800 50 55 55 (UK), International, +44 (0) 1382 800 50 55 55
* Beauty Bible, for information on beauty and beauty products:
www.beautybible.com
* Benefit, tel: +1 800 781 2336,
www.benefitcosmetics.com
* Birkenstock,
tel: +44 (0) 800 132 194,
www.birkenstock.com
* Bobbi Brown,
tel: +44 (0) 1730 232 566,
www.bobbibrowncosmetics.com
* Boots the chemist,
tel: +44 (0) 845 070 8090,
www.wellbeing.com
* Botanical Therapeutics, at Victoria Health, tel: 0800 389 8195, International, +44 1733 709 100,
www.victoriahealth.com

C

* Chanel,
tel: +44 (0) 20 7493 3836,
www.chanel.com
* Clinique,
tel: +44 (0) 1730 232 566,
www.clinique.com
* Coconut oil from some supermarkets and online:
www.essenceofeden.co.uk
* Crème de la Mer,
tel: +44 (0) 1730 232 566,
www.cremedelamer.com

D

* Dead Sea bath crystals, by Ahava, available at Victoria Health (see above)
* Dermablend,
tel: +44 (0) 2476 644 356,
www.dermablend.com
* Dermanova Products:
www.wellcene.co.uk
* Diana B, tel: +1 310 470 1170,
www.dianabbeauty.com

* Dr Lipp, tel: +44 (0) 20 7499 0163,
www.drlipp.com
* Dr Nick Lowe,
tel: +44 (0) 20 7499 3223,
available at Boots, www.boots.com
* Dr Scholl's,
tel: +1 866 360 3226,
www.drscholls.com

E

* Earth Naturals,
tel: +1 734 786 1531,
www.earthsoap.com
* Ecover,
tel: +44 (0) 8451 30 22 30,
www.ecover.com
* Ecozone wash balls,
tel: +44 (0) 845 230 4200,
www.ecozone.co.uk
* Eczema, clothing for babies and children, by Little Protechtor,
tel: +44 (0) 114 249 0603,
www.little-protechtor.com
* Equazen,
tel: +44 (0) 870 241 5621,
www.equazen.com
* Essie, tel: +1 718 726 5000,
www.essie.com
* Estée Lauder,
tel: +44 (0) 1730 232 566,
www.esteelauder.com
* Exercise balls, BUPA online shop,
tel: +44 (0) 1784 466 188,
www.shop.bupa.com
* Exercise equipment,
tel: +1 864 346-0945,
www.ballsnbands.com
* Exercise, fitness instructor, Viv Worrall, www.bodyandself.co.uk
* Eylure,
tel: +44 (0) 20 8573 9907,
www.eylure.com

F

* Fish from sustainable sources – Marine Conservation Society: www.fishonline.org
* FlitFlop, tel: +44 (0) 207 937 7887,
www.theflitflop.com
* Foam rollers,
tel: +44 (0) 1775 640 972,
www.physiosupplies.com

G

* Giorgio Armani,
www.giorgioarmanibeauty.com
* Guerlain, tel: +44 (0) 1932 233 874, www.guerlain.com

H

* Household cleaners (natural)
BioD, tel: +44 (0) 1482 229950,

www.biodegradable.biz

J

* Jekka's herb books,
tel: +44 (0) 1454 418 878,
www.jekkasherbfarm.com

K

* Kanebo, tel: +44 (0) 1635 46362,
www.kanebo-cosmetics.com
* Kerry September,
tel: +44 (0) 7748 594 442,
www.kerryseptember.com

L

* Lancôme, www.lancome.com
* Laura Mercier,
tel: +1 888 637 2437,
www.lauramercier.com
* Leighton Denny,
tel: +44 (0) 845 8620 515,
www.leightondenny.com
* Liz Earle Company details:
* Liz Earle by mail, (UK),
tel: + 44 1983 813939,
www.lizearle.com
* Liz Earle stores, (UK), Liz Earle Skincare and Treatment Rooms,
tel: 020 7881 7750
* Liz Earle Isle of Wight store, (Union, Isle of Wight),
tel: +44 (0) 1983 813913
* Liz Earle by mail, (Germany),
tel: +44 1983 813939,
www.lizearle.de
* Liz Earle by mail, (Republic of Ireland), tel: +44 1983 813939,
www.lizearle.ie
* Liz Earle by mail, (USA),
tel: +1 800 515 5911,
www.us.lizearle.com
* L'Oréal, tel: +44 (0) 800 072 6699,
www.loreal.com

M

* MAC Cosmetics,
tel: +44 (0) 20 7534 9222,
www.maccosmetics.com
* Max Factor, www.maxfactor.com
* Method, available at Boots and leading supermarkets,
tel: +44 (0) 845 070 8090,
www.methodproducts.com

N

* Nars, www.narscosmetics.co.uk
* Neck cushions,
tel: +44 (0) 1329 846273,
www.lavender-wheat-bags.co.uk
* Nelsons, tel: +44 (0) 20 8780 4200, www.nelsons.net
* Neutro Roberts,
tel: +39 800 827 176,

www.neutroroberts.it
* Nordic Walking,
tel: +44 (0) 845 260 9339,
www.nordicwalking.co.uk

O

* Origins, tel: +44 (0) 870 034 2949,
www.origins.com
* Opi, tel: +1 818 759 2400,
www.opi.com

P

* Pillows, Tempur,
tel: +44 (0) 8000 111 083,
www.tempur.com
* Prescriptives,
tel: +44 (0) 1730 232 566,
www.prescriptives.com

R

* Revital
+44 (0) 870 366 5729
www.revital.co.uk
* RMK, tel: at Selfridges,
+44 (0) 20 7318 3538,
www.rmkrmk.com
* Ruby and Millie, tel: at Boots,
+44 (0) 845 609 0055,
www.boots.com, see also: www.rubyandmillie.com

S

* Shu Uemura,
tel: +44 (0) 20 7379 6627,
www.shu-uemura.co.jp
* Solgar Vitamins,
tel: +44 (0) 1442 890355,
www.solgar.com
* Stila, tel: +44 (0) 1730 232 566,
www.stilacosmetics.com

T

* The Body Shop,
tel: +44 (0) 1903 844 554,
www.thebodyshop.com
* T-shirts: www.isiah61clothing.com

V

* Victoria Health
tel: +44 (0) 1733 709 100,
www.victoriahealth.com

W

* Weleda, tel: +44 (0) 115 9448 222,
www.weleda.com

X

* Xylitol, Perfect Sweet:
www.perfectsweet.co.uk
* Yves St Laurent,
tel: +44 (0) 1444 255 700,
www.ysl.com.

Glossary

Acid mantle – a very fine, slightly acidic film (a mix of sebum and sweat) on the skin surface which acts as a barrier to infections and invaders

Acne – a skin condition causing blocked and infected pores that result in blackheads and whiteheads, pimples and cysts, on the face, neck, chest, back, and shoulders

Adipose cells – 'adipocytes' store energy as fat

Adrenaline – also called epinephrine, a 'fight or flight' hormone produced in the adrenal glands when the body is under physical, mental or emotional stress

Alpha-spinasterol – a compound that stimulates cell regeneration

Amino-acids – the building blocks of protein, completely essential for our bodies to function; we can produce ten of the 20 amino acids; the others must come from food (meat, milk and eggs contain all the essential amino-acids, nuts, beans and soy beans have high levels) – they can't be stored, so a good diet is vital

Antioxidants: natural substances, including vitamins C and E, that help protect cells from 'oxidative stress' – damage caused by unstable molecules called free radicals

Apocrine gland – a sweat gland attached to hair follicles, mainly under the armpits and in the genital area

Arginine – a 'food source' for the virus that causes warts

Aromatherapy – a complementary therapy that uses fragrant essential oils and other aromatic compounds to affect mind and body; often combined with massage

Ayurvedic – the traditional medicine system of India: literally, the science (veda) of life (ayus) Basal layer – the bottom layer of the epidermis (top layer of the skin), where cells begin their lives

Benzophenone – a family of synthetic chemicals found in chemical sunscreens

Benzoyl peroxide – common ingredient in acne formulations which works by taking oxygen into the infected pores and killing the bacteria; however, it's very drying and may cause skin to overreact and produce more oil

Beta-carotene – a precursor of vitamin A

Biofeedback – a technique that helps control involuntary physical functions, such as breathing, heart rate and muscle contractions

Capillaries – the smallest blood vessels

Carcinogenic – any substance that is directly involved in the promotion or spread of cancer

Cardiovascular system – this consists of the heart and a closed system of vessels (arteries, veins and capillaries), which circulates blood around every cell of the body; often linked with the lymphatic system as 'the circulatory system'

Catechin – chemical found in black tea and dark chocolate

Cellulite – pockets of trapped fat found commonly on women's thighs and buttocks, which cause dimpling; occurs in 90 per cent of post-adolescent women, rare in men

Chlorella – single-celled green algae (marine plant), which contains high amounts of chlorophyll; can be dried as whole-food nutritional supplement

Chlorophyll – green pigment found in most plants and algae, which is vital for photosynthesis, the process by which plants obtain energy from light

Choline – trace element linked to improved brain function

Chromosomes – each cell contains 23 pairs of chromosones, which carry DNA (see below) and tell the cell what to do

Cinnamate – a family of synthetic chemicals found in chemical sunscreens

Citral – chemical component of natural essential oils

Citronellol – chemical perfumery constituent

Collagen – the largest part of the skin's support structure, found particularly in the dermis, together with elastin fibres: gives skin its resilience, tone and stretch

Connective tissue – a type of tissue (group of cells) made up of fibres that form a framework and support structure for body tissues and organs. In skin terms, the most important fibres are made up of collagen and elastin

Corneocytes – flattened-out cells in the top horny layer (stratum corneum) of the epidermis (top layer of skin)

Cortisol – a corticosteroid hormone produced by the adrenal glands, involved in the stress response; cortisol rises naturally in the early morning to increase blood pressure and blood sugar in preparation for the day

Cortisone – a type of hormone/steroid-like compound that acts to quell inflammation; however, cortisone creams may thin the skin, long term

Delta 7 stigmasterol – a compound that stimulates cell regeneration

Dihydroxyacetone – synthetic molecule, principle ingredient in self-tanners

Dermatitis – any inflamed red skin condition, including eczema and psoriasis

Dermis – the second layer of skin, under the epidermis

Desquamation – the skin's natural exfoliation process, in which the top dead cells of the epidermis are sloughed off

DNA – stands for deoxyribonucleic acid, the famous double helix that contains the genetic instructions used in the development and functioning of all known living organisms

Eccrine gland – a type of sweat gland, responsible for most of the body's sweat output and found all over the body

Eicosapentanoic acid (EPA) – one of the omega-3 polyunsaturated essential fatty acids; the others are alpha-linolenic acid (ALA) and docosahexanoic acid (DHA)

Eczema – inflammation of the epidermis, a form of dermatitis

EFAs – essential fatty acids, the fats or lipids that provide the building blocks of healthy skin, and play a significant role in the structure and function of every cell; they are essential, but the body can't manufacture them, so they have to be derived from diet; often referred to as omega-3s and 6s

Elastin – a protein in connective tissue that is elastic and allows skin to bounce back after stretching or contracting

Emollients – substances that soften and soothe the skin, used to correct dryness and scaling

Epidermis – the surface layer of skin

Essential fatty acids – see EFAs

Exfoliate – to remove the top dead layer of cells on the skin surface, revealing fresh skin underneath

Follicle – a very fine tube opening on the surface of the skin, which may or may not contain a hair

Formaldehyde – a potentially toxic chemical ingredient which is a common ingredient in nail polish (as a hardener), classified as a probable human carcinogen by the US Environmental Protection Agency

Free radicals – unpaired molecules that damage cells in their search for a mate, principally through a process called oxidative stress; free radicals can be neutralised by antioxidants

Gernaoil – chemical perfumery constituent

GLA – gamma-linolenic acid, an omega-6 essential fatty acid found principally in plant-based oils such as evening primrose and borage

Glucosamine – provides the building blocks to repair connective tissue

Glycaemic Index (GI) – a measure of the effects of carbohydrates (starches and sugars) on the sugar (glucose) levels in the blood; high-GI foods release sugar (as glucose) rapidly into the bloodstream, while low-GI foods initiate a slower process

Glycaemic Load – similar to the GI, but allows a more precise measurement of the carbohydrates in a food and how they affect your blood sugar levels

Glycation – process where a sugar molecule bonds to a protein or lipid (fat) molecule without being controlled by an enzyme, which may, among other things, degrade collagen, causing wrinkles

Hormones – the body's chemical messengers, which transport signals from one cell to another; they're involved in virtually everything we do, from sleep to reproduction to appetite

Human chorionic gonadtrophin (HCG) – pregnancy hormone

Hydrocortisone – treats inflammation but blocks wound healing

Hypodermis – subcutaneous layer of skin

Hyaluronic acid – aka hyaluronate, hyaluronon; a major component of skin, where it is involved in tissue repair; also vital in synovial fluid, which lubricates joints, and many other functions

Hydrogenation – forcing hydrogen at high pressure and temperature into liquid oils to prevent them becoming solid at room temperature; it results in a mixture of unnatural fats, many of which are trans fatty acids (transfats), known to be dangerous to the heart and possibly linked to certain cancers

Hypothyroidism – condition where the thyroid gland produces insufficient thyroxin hormone to keep the body functioning properly, causing muscle weakness, fatigue, dry flaky skin, weight gain

Iodine – trace element required for thyroid hormone

Keratinocytes – skin cells; keratin is the protein in skin, hair and nails

Kigelinone – active compound of the napthoquinone group, with anti-inflammatory properties

Langerhans cells – immune cells found in the epidermis (top layer of skin)

Linalool – chemical component of natural essential oils

Linoleic acid – an essential fatty acid found principally in plant-based oils such as borage

Lipids – fats

Lymph – clear yellowish fluid that flows round the body, sweeping up threatening substances, eg, toxins, bacteria and viruses

Lymphatic system – network of fine, fluid-filled tubes and small glands (nodes) that runs throughout the body, operating in tandem with your blood circulation (see Lymph, above)

Melanin – pigment that controls your skin colour, how much you tan, your hair colour, and helps protect your skin against sunlight

Melanocytes – pigment cells

Melanoma – malignant melanoma is a rare but potentially fatal form of skin cancer, involving melanocytes (see above); basal cell and squamous cell carcinomas are common, but much less serious forms of skin tumours, categorised as 'non-melanoma' skin cancers

Melatonin – sleep hormone

Metabolism – the chemical reactions that occur in living organisms in order to maintain life; metabolites are products of metabolism

Methyl paraben – a naturally occurring paraben found particularly in vanilla pods

Monounsaturated fats – fats such as olive oil that are typically liquid at room temperature and start to solidify when chilled; usually high in vitamin E and, eaten in reasonable amounts, beneficial for health

Naturopathy – a form of complementary alternative medicine which heals the body holistically

Neuropeptides – the brain chemicals released into the nerve endings triggered by psychological stress

Non-acnegenic – a name for products aimed at those with acne which has no legal definition

NMF – Natural Moisturising Factor: a group of chemicals in the skin which act like a magnet for water

Non-comedogenic – not likely to block pores in most people

Octyl salicylate – a type of synthetic sunscreen

Oestrogen – the female reproductive hormone

Omega-3 and -6 – see essential fatty acids

Osteoporosis – loss of bone mineral density, leading to thinner bones more prone to fracture

Oxidation – oxidative stress – the cell-damaging process caused by free radicals; antioxidants counter it

Parabens – family of preservatives

pH balance – the acid/alkaline balance of the skin, which ranges from 0, the most acid, to 14, the most alkaline; normal skin is 5.5. Products labelled pH balanced have been formulated to have a pH close to that

Phenol – an antioxidant found in black tea and dark chocolate

Phenoxyethanol – an effective preservative used in face creams

Phenylethyl – chemical perfumery constituent

Phospholipids – fatty acids that form the 'cement' of the skin barrier and come under attack by free radicals

Phyto-oestrogens – oestrogens (estrogens), natural reproductive hormones, derived from plant (phyto-) sources

Phytosterols – plant-derived fatty molecules with a similar structure to skin sterols (fats or lipids) and also cholesterol; used in moisturisers to restore and rejuvenate skin

Phytotherapy – the use of plants or plant extracts medicinally

Pilates – exercise method focusing on building your body's core strength and improving posture through low-impact stretching and conditioning exercises

Pityriasis capitis – the Latin name for common dandruff meaning 'scaly head'

Polyphenol compounds – antioxidants derived from plants such as aloe vera

Pores – where follicles (see left) open on the skin's surface

Probiotics – dietary supplements containing 'good' bacteria for the gut, which help support health in many ways; often recommended after a course of antibiotics, which diminishes 'good' as well as 'bad' bugs in the gut

Procollagen – a precursor (forerunner) of collagen

Progesterone – one of the two main female reproductive hormones; the other is oestrogen

Propylene glycol – a potential skin irritant in high doses, though in small doses has softening and emollient properties

Psoriasis – non-contagious, inflammatory skin disease caused by speeded-up cell growth and excessive shedding

Reactive oxygen species (ROS) – the collective term for oxygen free radicals (see above), the type that cause most problems for our body cells

Rosacea – chronic skin disease which typically causes flushing and redness over the centre of the face

Salicylic acid – a beta-hydroxy acid derived from the bark of the willow tree (Salix), used to clear and prevent blackheads and pimples

Sebum – oily substance produced by the sebaceous glands in the skin

Selenium – an important antioxidant found in chicken eggs

Sodium lauryl sulfates (SLS) or sodium laureth sulfates (SLES) – a commonly used detergent, and well-known skin irritant that can thin the skin barrier. Bad reaction can include redness, itchiness, burning and stinging

Solar keratoses – small, rough, slightly raised bumps, ranging from the size of a pinhead to two or three centimetres across, usually on the face, neck, backs of hands, bald patch and other areas often exposed to the sun – a warning sign that skin has been under sun assault

Staphylococcus aureus – a bacterium that lives in the nose and gets into the hair follicles after shaving, potentially causing barber's rash

Steroid – topical steroids, aka corticosteroids, are used to treat inflammatory skin conditions, including eczema

Sterols – found in plants and help to reduce age spots, sun damage and scars

Stratum corneum – the top surface layer of the epidermis, also known as the horny layer, which is composed of dead cells called corneocytes

Subcutaneous – just under the skin

T-zone – oily patch across the forehead and down the nose to chin

Teripen-4-ol – an antibacterial found in tea tree oil

Testosterone – one of the reproductive hormones; the dominant hormone in men but women have some, too; the ratio of oestrogen to testosterone changes with menopause, as oestrogen declines and the relative level of testosterone goes up

TEWL – Trans Epidermal Water Loss, which occurs if the skin barrier (the stratum corneum) is damaged, allowing fluid to escape; high TEWL is linked to increased permeability, allowing infections and irritants to get through the barrier

Titanium – mineral found in mineral sunscreen (together with zinc oxide)

Transfats – trans fatty acids formed by hydrogenating liquid fats (see hydrogenation)

Trans-retinoic acid – a form of vitamin A which helps remove the top dead layer of skin cells

Triterpernoids – an extract found in Calendula which is said to have antiseptic and healing properties, that prevent the spread of infection and speed up the rate of repair

UVA, UVB and UVC – the wavelengths of sunlight, aka UV light; most UVC – the shortest wavelength – is filtered out by the atmosphere, but UVA (the longest) and UVB radiation both reach the earth in significant amounts. UVA penetrates deep into the skin, causing ageing; UVB burns the epidermis. Both can cause skin cancer

Xanthine oxidase – an enzyme that, undigested, attacks the arterial walls and parts of the heart muscle, causing inflammation

Zeaxanthine – a skin-supporting antioxidant found in organic milk

Zinc oxide – mineral found in mineral sunscreen (together with titanium)

Organisations

Acne:
* British Association of Dermatologists tel:+44 (0) 20 7383 0266,
* www.bad.org.uk See also, Herbalists, for: National Institute of Medical Herbalists and Register of Chinese Herbal Medicine.
* Factsheet from www.lizearle.com

Acupuncture:
* Acupuncture Association (SA), tel: +27 (0) 31 205 8845, www.physiosa.org.za
* Australian Acupuncture and Chinese Medicine Association, tel: +61 (0) 7 3324 2599, www.acupuncture.org.au
* British Acupuncture Council, tel: +44 (0) 20 8735 0400, www.acupuncture.org.uk
* Chinese Medicine and Acupuncture Association of Canada, tel: +1 519 642 1970, www.cmaac.ca
* New Zealand Register of Acupuncturists Inc, tel: +64 (0) 4 387 7672, www.acupuncture.org.nz
* Singapore Acupuncture Association, tel: +65 63 545760, www.acupuncture.org.sg

Allergies:
* Allergy Society of South Africa, tel: +27 (0) 21 447 9019, www.allergysa.org
* Allergy UK, tel: +44 (0) 1322 619898, www.allergyuk.org
* Australasian Society of Clinical Immunology and Allergy, www.allergy.org.au
* Canadian Society of Allergy and Clinical Immunology, tel: +1 613 730 6272, www.csaci.ca
* Singapore Association of Rheumatology, Allergy and Immunology, tel: +65 63 577822, www.aar.clinic.com

Aromatherapy:
* Aromatherapy Associates, (UK), tel: +44 (0) 20 8567 2243, www.aromatherapyassociates.com
* Aromatherapy Society of South Africa, tel: +27 (0)826677746, www.asosa.org.za
* Australian Aromatic Medicine Association Inc, tel: +61 (0) 3 9016 0600, www.aama-oz.org
* Canadian Federation of Aromatherapists, tel: +1 519 746 1594 www.cfacanada.com
* Cancer information, (UK), Breakthrough Breast Cancer, tel: +44 (0) 20 7025 2400, www.breakthrough.co.uk
* Cosmetic Toiletry and Perfumery Association UK:

www.thefactsabout.co.uk
* International Federation of Aromatherapists, tel: +44 (0) 20 8567 2243, www.ifparoma.org
* New Zealand Register of Holistic Aromatherapists, www.aromatherapy.org.nz
* Singapore Physiotherapy Association: www.physiotherapy.org.sg

Dermatology:
* Australasian College of Dermatologists, tel: +61 (0) 2 8765 0242, or 1300 361 821, (Australia only), www.dermcoll.asn.au
* British Association of Dermatologists, (Acne factsheet), tel: +44 (0) 20 7383 0266, www.bad.org.uk
* Canadian Dermatology Association, tel: +1 613 738 1748, www.dermatology.ca
* Dermatological Society of Singapore, tel: +65 91 294583, www.dermatology.org.sg
* Dermnet (NZ Dermatological Society): www.dermnet.org.nz

Eczema:
* Allergy Society of South Africa, tel: +27 (0) 21 447 9019, www.allergysa.org
* Eczema Association of Australasia Inc., tel: +61 (0) 7 3206 3633, or 1300 300 182, (Australia only), www.eczema.org.au
* Eczema information website: www.undermyskin.co.uk
* Eczema Society of Canada, tel: +1 905 535 0776, www.eczemahelp.ca
* European Cosmetic Toiletry and Perfumery Association, which contains useful information on EU legislation and product labeling: www.colipa.com
* National Eczema Society (UK), (Eczema factsheet), tel: +44 (0) 800 089 1122, www.eczema.org
* National Skin Centre, (Singapore), tel: +65 62 534455, www.nsc.gov.sg
* Factsheet from www.lizearle.com

Herbalists:
* The Canadian Association of Naturopathic Doctors, tel: +1 416 496 8633, www.naturopathicassoc.ca
* Herbal Practitioners South Africa, email via website, www.herbalpractitionerssa.co.za
* National Herbalists Association of Australia, tel: +61 (0) 2 8765 0071, www.nhaa.org.au
* National Institute of Medical

Herbalists, (UK), tel: +44 (0) 1392 426022, www.nimh.org.uk
* New Zealand Association of Medical Herbalists, email: info@nzamh.org.nz, www.nzamh.org.nz
* Register of Chinese Herbal Medicine, (UK), tel: +44 (0) 1603 623 994, www.rchm.co.uk
* Society of Traditional Chinese Medicine, Singapore, tel: +65 63 230898, www.society-tcms.org

Homeopaths:
* Australian Homeopathic Association, tel: +61 (0) 3 5979 1558, www.homeopathyoz.org
* Homeopathic Association of South Africa: www.hsa.org.za
* Kidshealth, general information on child health: www.kidshealth.org
* New Zealand Homeopathic Society, tel: +64 (0) 9 630 5458, www.homeopathy.ac.nz
* Singapore Faculty of Homeopaths, tel: +65 62 994502, www.singaporehomeopathy.com
* Society of Homeopaths, (UK), tel: +44 (0) 845 450 6611, www.homeopathy-soh.org
* Factsheet from www.lizearle.com

Massage:
* Australian Association of Massage Therapists Ltd, tel: +61 (0) 3 9691 3700, or 1300 138 872 (Australia only), www.aamt.com
* Canadian Massage Therapists Alliance, tel: +1 604 873 4467, www.cmta.ca
* General Council for Massage Therapies, (UK), tel: +44 (0) 870 850 4452. www.gcmt.org.uk
* Manual Lymphatic Drainage, MLDUK, tel: +44 (0) 844 800 1988, www.mlduk.org.uk
* Massage New Zealand, tel: +64 (0) 9 623 8269, www.assagenewzealand.org
* Massage Therapy Association of South Africa, tel: +27 (0) 21 713 3006, www.mtasa.co.za
* Singapore Physiotherapy Association:www.physiotherapy.org.sg

Nutritional therapy:
* Association for Dietetics in South Africa, tel: +27 (0) 11 447 4187, www.dietetics.co.za
* British Association for Nutritional Therapy, tel: +44 (0) 870 606 1284, www.bant.org.uk
* Nutrition Society of Australia, tel: +61 (0) 8 8363 1307, www.nsa.asn.au
* Nutrition Society of New Zealand,

tel: +64 (0) 6 350 5962, www.nutritionsociety.ac.nz
* Singapore Nutrition and Dietetics Association: www.snda.org.sg

Osteopathy:
* European School of Osteopaths, tel: +44 (0) 1622 671558, www.eso.ac.uk
* General Osteopathic Council (UK), tel: +44 (0) 20 7357 6655, www.osteopathy.org
* World Osteopathic Health Organisation: www.woho.org

Psoriasis:
* Psoriatic Arthropathy Alliance, tel: + 44 (0) 870 770 3212, www.paalliance.org
* The Psoriasis Association, (Psoriasis factsheet), tel: +44 (0) 845 676 0076, www.psoriasis-association.org.uk
* Factsheet from www.lizearle.com

Reflexology:
* British Reflexology Association, tel: +44 (0) 1886 821207, www.britreflex.co.uk
* Reflexology Association of Australia, tel: +61 (0) 7 3396 9001, www.reflexology.org.au
* Reflexology Association of Canada, tel: +1 204 477 4909, www.reflexologycanada.ca
* Reflexology New Zealand: www.reflexology.org.nz
* South African Reflexology Society: www.sareflexology.org.za

Rosacea:
* Acne Rosacea Factsheet, (UK), Skincare Physicians: www.skincarephysicians.com/rosaceanet
* Dr Nase: www.drnase.com
* Institute of Trichologists, (international) tel: +44 (0) 870 607 0602, www.trichologists.org.uk
* Skin Care Campaign, tel: +44 (0) 20 7281 3553, www.skincarecampaign.org
* Soil Association, tel: +44 (0) 117 314 5000, www.soilassociation.org
* UK charity for scientific information written by leading scientists: www.senseaboutscience.org.uk
* Factsheet from www.lizearle.com

Yoga:
* Australian Institute of Yoga Therapy, tel: +61 (0) 3 59 68 1811, www.australian-institute-yoga.com.au
* British Wheel of Yoga, tel: +44 (0) 1529 306851, www.bwy.org.uk
* International Yoga Federation, www.internationalyogafederation.net
* Yoga Online, (NZ), tel: +64 (0) 6 751 1163, www.yoga.org.nz

Supplements and natural remedies

Here are details of the supplements with suggested brands I mention in the book. Most of the products are available online with free UK postage from www.victoriahealth.com Another useful website is www.revital.co.uk

VERY IMPORTANT: Always follow manufacturers recommendations for dosage and when to take. If you are pregnant, have a medical condition or taking pharmaceutical medicines, please consult your doctor first.

Chapter 3

Vitamin A by HealthAid; maintains a healthy outer skin layer (has helped PCOS sufferers with intractable acne).

Vitamin C with minerals will help maintain the collagen network; try Ester-C Plus by Solgar, or Emergen-C sachets by Alacer Corp when travelling.

Antioxidants:
These help protect the skin against free radical damage. Good products include: Advanced Antioxidant Formula by Solgar Vitamins; VM75 by Solgar Vitamins; GliSODin by Pure ZP, with superoxidedismutase (SOD).

Calcium and magnesium for healthy bones; try Bone Restore by Life Extension, for easily absorbed calcium together with magnesium, D3 and boron. Take minerals with your evening meal or before bed.

Chasteberry (agnus castus) by HealthAid; relieves muscle cramps, regulates hormone levels and menstrual cycles. Good for symptoms of PMS and menopause.

Chlorella, a freshwater green algae, has skin-nourishing properties and de-acidifies the gut; try Sun Chlorella A by Sun Chlorella. Take 15-40 tablets per day (start at the lower dose and increase gradually).

Colloidal silver by Source Naturals; apply directly to spots, or mix a few drops with your daily moisturiser to help keep your skin clear.

Digestive enzymes:
Try ExtraZyme 13 by Lifetime Vitamins, before each meal. For further colon cleansing, try Fibre FOS and Acidophilus by Nutrition Now.

Essential fatty acids:
Essential Oil Formula by Harmony Formula: a blend of omega-3, 6, 9.
Omega 3-6-9 Softgels by Solgar Vitamins: a blend of oils from fish, flax and borage oils.
   Eye Q, capsules or liquid, by Equazen: with fish oil and evening primrose oil.
   Organic Omega 3:6:9 Balance Oil

(liquid form) by Higher Nature
   Organic Ultimate Beauty Oil (liquid) by Viridian Nutrition: this gives you omega-3, 6 and 9, plus a broad range of antioxidants.
Ester-E by Lifetime Vitamins; for small sun or 'age' spots on your face, split capsule and massage on face with a little rosehip oil.
Pure Hyaluronic Acid by Syno-Vital (one of the few vegetarian HA products) helps lubricate joints and skin.
Phyto-estrogens help balance hormones and protect the skin against premature ageing; try Ladies Choice, combines pomegranate seed, offering an abundant source of phyto-oestrogen, with soya isoflavones and other important ingredients intended to provide support for physical and emotional well-being during midlife.
Xylitol is an ideal natural sweetener found in fruit and plants for people wanting to avoid sugar; it's been shown to strengthen bones and teeth and is suitable for diabetics; try Perfect Sweet.
Zinc with Copper by Natures Own; to help heal acne and prevent scarring.

Chapter 4

Cellulite products:
Horse Chestnut reduces excess tissue fluid and protects capillaries; try Aesculus Forte by BioForce (A. Vogel).
Ester C by Lamberts Vitamins delivers higher vitamin C levels inside the cells.
Vitamin E improves circulation and is necessary for tissue repair; try Ester-E by Lifetime Vitamins.
Gingko Biloba increases peripheral circulation and tissue oxygenation; try Quest Vitamins.
Glucosamine Sulphate (try Lamberts) has a role in strengthening cellular membranes so that cells don't dehydrate.
Bioflavonoids help prevent the migration of wasted water outside skin cells which can result in the dimpling effect; try Citrus Bioflavonoids by Solgar Vitamins.
Butcher's Broom (by Nature's Way) contains active ruscogenin.
Iron supplements:
   Spatone, by Spatone, is a natural iron food; or try Floradix by Salus, which provides organic iron.
   Magnesium may improve nail health; try Dyno-Mins by Nature's Plus.
Silica helps promote healthy hair, skin and nails; try Silica 2500 Plus by Kordels.

Chapter 5

Vitamin D3 (by Lifetime Vitamins) is

increasingly recognised as an important supplement; helps build healthy bones and reduces the risk of osteoporosis and other diseases.

Chapter 6

Probiotics support the digestive system, increasing energy and improving metabolism; try Mega-Probiotic-ND by Food Sciences of Vermont.
Zinc is an important anti-inflammatory mineral present in all body tissues, crucial to numerous body functions; try Zinc Picolinate by Lifetime Vitamins.

Natural Prescription: Eczema
✳ Blood purifying herbs such as red clover, dandelion, burdock, sarsaparilla help reduce skin inflammation; try Red Clover Combination by Doctor's A-Z.
✳ Essential Fatty Acids (EFA's) help restore the skin's lipid levels to prevent flaking and dry skin: try Essential Oil Formula by Harmony Formula, containing omega-3, 6 and 9; for a vegetarian version derived from algae, try V-Pure Omega-3 by Water4life (www.water4.net); hemp seed, flaxseed and evening primrose oil are all good sources of EFAs, found in Ultimate Beauty Oil by Viridian Nutrition.
✳ Biotin deficiency: try a good B complex supplement such as Vitamin B50 by Lifetime Vitamins.
✳ Topical creams to help prevent itching: try Skin Cream Plus by Botanical Therapeutics, Botanical Shampoo and Botanical Conditioner, also by Botanical Therapeutics, may help alleviate inflammatory scalp problems. (Leave them on for a few minutes to allow the ingredients to work effectively.)
✳ Medihoney moisturising cream, by Medihoney is an excellent cream based on medicinal honey.
✳ Oat based products help soothe eczema and other inflammatory skin conditions: try Aveeno Eczema Care cream by Johnson and Johnson (www.aveeno.co.uk).
✳ 2 per cent licorice products help reduce redness, swelling and itching: try Hope's Relief Cream by Hope's (www.hopesrelief.co.uk). Licorice based products can also help cold sores: try Lomabrit by Britannia Health or Spot On by Liz Earle.

Natural Prescription: Psoriasis
✳ Liver cleanse: try Ultimate Liver Cleanse by Nature's Secret, which combines milk thistle, dandelion root and artichoke leaf extract to cleanse and support the liver.
✳ Vitamin A by HealthAid

✳ Vitamin D3 by Lifetime Vitamins
✳ Essential Fatty Acids
✳ Zinc Picolinate by Lifetime Vitamins
✳ Lactoferrin, a bovine protein, has been shown to calm psoriasis (and acne): try Lactoferrin by Southern Country
✳ Red Clover Combination by Doctor's A-Z (see Eczema)
✳ Sun Chlorella A by Sun Chlorella.
✳ Herbal teas help cleanse the body and soothe skin; try Skin Purify Tea by Dr Stuart, with red clover, nettles and lemon balm.
✳ Topical emollients with ceramides may help repair skin barrier: try Aveeno Eczema Care cream by Johnson and Johnson (www.aveeno.co.uk), as for eczema; Calendula Cream by HealthAid; CerVe by Coria (www.cerave.com); Mimyx cream by Stiefel (www.mimyx.com); Aloe Vera HP Cream by HealthAid.

Natural Prescription: Acne
✳ Vitamin A by HealthAid
✳ Vitamin D3 by Lifetime Vitamins
✳ Zinc Picolinate by Lifetime Vitamins
✳ Essential Fatty Acids
✳ ActivClear cream by Nutrica, with Tea Tree Oil.
✳ Cholayil Pvt. Ltd may help remove impurities in the blood that cause pimples, blackheads, boils, acne, cysts, spots and other skin problems.
✳ Lactoferrin, a bovine protein, has been shown to calm acne (and psoriasis): try Lactoferrin by Southern Country.

Natural prescription: Rosacea
✳ Essential Fatty Acids: try Ultimate Beauty Oil by Viridian (see Eczema)
✳ Probiotics: try Mega-Probiotic-ND by Food Sciences of Vermont
✳ Digestive enzymes: try Extrazyme 13 by Lifetime Vitamins
✳ Cream containing *Chrysanthellum indicum*: try Phytomer Douceur Marine Velvety Soothing Cream by Phytomer (www.phytomer.fr)
✳ Cream containing green tea: try Alpha Lipoic - Green Tea Cream by Derma E skin care
✳ Cream containing 2 per cent licorice: try Hope's Relief Cream by Hope's (www.hopesrelief.co.uk)
✳ Cream containing Azelaic acid: try Skinoren Cream by Valeant (www.valeant.com)
✳ Pycnogenol Redness Reducing Serum by Derma E contains an extract from the pine bark tree which has a powerful anti-inflammatory effect.
✳ MSM Cream by At Last Naturals contains organic sulphur (sulphur was used in the Victorian era for rosacea

Index

Dedicated to
Four children and Mad Ox

This paperback edition published in Great Britain in 2011 by
Kyle Books
23 Howland Street, London, W1T 4AY
www.kylebooks.com

First published in hardback in Great Britain in 2009 by Kyle Cathie Limited

ISBN: 978-0-85783-030-2

A CIP catalogue record for this title is available from the British Library

Photography acknowledgements:
Special photography by Patrick Drummond: jacket, pp. 1, 2, 4–9, 11, 12, 14, 15, 16, 17, 24–5, 26, 30, 35, 36, 38–9, 44–5, 61, 63, 82–3, 93, 95, 104–5, 106–7, 108, 110, 111, 113, 114, 116–7, 119, 123, 124, 127, 139, 146, 157, 160–1, 162, 174–5, 178, 180–1, 192

Special Photography by Kate Whitaker: pp. 21, 23, 47–58, 62, 66–75, 79–81, 84–91, 94, 96, 99–103, 121, 128, 131–7, 141–5, 150–6, 159, 13–172

Photography on pp.16-17: far right, 2nd row, Camera Press; 2nd from left and 2nd from the right, 3rd row: Jupiter Images; p.76: Getty Images

Design: Dale Walker
Photography: Patrick Drummond and Kate Whitaker
Illustrations: Kathy Wyatt
Editor: Sophie Allen
Copy editor: Simon Canney
Props stylist: Ali Allen (chapter 7)
Food stylist: Annie Nichols (on pp. 121, chapter 7)
Hair and make-up: Kerry September (front jacket, pp. 11, 12, 15, 106, 146, 178, 180-1)
Hair and make-up: Craig Beaglehole (pp. 6, 61)
Hair: Andreas at John Freida (pp. 47, 48, 66, 70)
Make up: Nicky Weir (pp. 47, 48, 66, 70)
Hair and make-up: Marie Coulter (pp. 50, 52, 53, 55-8, 75, 79, 163-172)
Production: Sha Huxtable

Razor used on p. 81 courtesy of Geo. F. Trumper
Clothes used on pp. 57, 68 courtesy of The White Company

Printed and bound in China by 1010 Printing International Ltd.

Acknowledgements:
Ali Allen, Sophie Allen, Ann Bawtree, David Bawtree, Craig Beaglehole, Dr Mabel Blades, Liz Bonser, Hilary Boyd, Kim Buckland, Caroline Burnstein-Collis, Kyle Cathie, Professor Charles Clarke, Andrew Chevallier, Professor Michael Cork, Marie Coulter, Sarah Daw, Shabir Daya , Fiona Dowal, Patrick Drummond, Pauline Dunmore, Guy Earle, Lily Earle, Francesca Forman, Alex Marx, Louise Mackaness, Delphine Gaborit, Jo Givens, Professor Jonathan Hadgraft, Tracy Hastain, Liz Hellyer, Jennifer Hirsch, Amy Holliday, Toni Jade, Arezoo Kaviani, Andry Kirlappou, Hannah Lovegrove, Felicity Lyons, Oliver Lyons, Anna Macleod, Tom Mammone, Neil McCall, Sam Middleton, Dr Georges Mouton, Louise Murray, Sarah Newton, Dr David Orentreich, Robertet, Raquel Santos , Kerry September, Steve Simmonds, Wei Tang, Kate Todd, Dr Ann Walker, Dale Walker, Owen Walker, Nicky Weir, Kate Whitaker, Andreas Wild, Viv Worrall

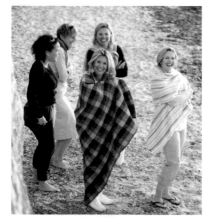

It's a wrap!
Left to right: Kerry, Sarah, Kim, Tracy (and Liz)
Thank you